DYING

AND

LIVING

ON

THE

KANSAS

PRAIRIE

A Diary

Carol Brunner Rutledge

University Press of Kansas

DYING

AND

LIVING

ON

THE

KANSAS

PRAIRIE

A Diary

© 1994 by the University Press of Kansas

Published by the University Press of Kansas (Lawrence, Kansas 66049),
which was organized by the Kansas Board of Regents and is operated
and funded by Emporia State University, Fort Hays State University,
Kansas State University, Pittsburg State University, the University of
Kansas, and Wichita State University

Library of Congress Cataloging-in-Publication Data

Rutledge, Carol Brunner
Dying and living on the Kansas prairie: a diary /
Carol Brunner Rutledge
p.   cm.
ISBN 0-7006-0649-1 (alk. paper)
1. Brunner, Alice—Health. 2. Mitral valve prolapse—
Displacement—Patients—Kansas—Biography.
3. Women—Kansas—Biography.   I. Title.
RC685.V2B787   1994
362.1'75—dc20
[B]   94-13492

British Library Cataloging in Publication Data is available.

Printed in the United States of America

10 9 8 7 6 5 4 3 2 1

The paper used in this publication meets
the minimum requirements of the American
National Standard for Permanence of Paper for
Printed Library Materials Z39.48-1984.

FOR

JOHN

AND

HELEN

DYING

AND

LIVING

ON

THE

KANSAS

PRAIRIE

A Diary

THE END

I don't know when I first decided to keep a diary of her dying. I don't know why it seemed important to do so. But one day at the beginning of that very different summer, I looked at Mother and thought, "This is going to happen to me someday." So I started to take notes. What was seen, what was said, and how it fit into the prairie around us. When it was over, I had a log of her dying. And my healing.

As we floated through the haze of those ninety days, feelings were sometimes heightened and illuminated, sometimes shadowed and conflicted. It was a time spent balancing our tremendous need for the medical profession with their refusal to acknowledge Mother's most important need— support for her spirit while her body died.

Now, and for the rest of my life, I will remember the three months she lay there surrounded by people who had not come to their own understanding of death. From silent body language to the deceptive "You must eat, Alice, so you can get well and go home," they tried to control her dying. She never wavered in her faith, and she ended life the way she had lived: with laughter and with love.

ON THE
PRE-AGRARIAN
PRAIRIE

(Before Europeans Came)

First Scene

The wind is twin to the sun on the rolling prairie. In winter, it blows straight down from the snow plains. In summer it sweeps up from the land of red earth.

It dives and twists across the grasslands while bison huddle in low areas, massive heads facing the onslaught. Tall grasses wrench back and forth and swirl.

Just as suddenly, the wind is still. There is no motion. Then comes a rustle in the grass, a warbling bird song. Slowly, prairie creatures resume their ways. Wind is the only force that can command such an abrupt break in life. It will return.

FROM THE DIARY
IN JUNE

June 19

Looking at nothing.

The call I was expecting from my sister came early today.
"We took Mother to the hospital again." Helen's voice
sounded strained and sad, and there was a moment of silence
between us. We both realized it would probably be the last
trip for Mother to the little hospital that our family has used
for generations. There she will be cared for by neighbors
who call each other by first name and who love our Mother,
as she loves them.

Now, with a thermos of coffee beside me in our four-wheel
drive, my sunglasses waiting on the dash, the air conditioner
on, and the gas tank full, I face this long Kansas road again.

Between my home in Topeka on the eastern edge of the
Flint Hills and Hope on the western side, there are a hundred
miles of prairie and sky. This tall-grass land has sheltered
my people for generations. It has taunted us and calmed us,
broken us and nurtured us, starved us and fed us. It is our
span over birth, growth, and death. Death, which beckons
now to my Mother.

Now I drive down the purple hills where the grass stretches beyond the horizon. I once asked three-year-old Tahne what she sees here.

> "Grass and sky."
> "What else?"
> "Nothing."
> "How do you look at nothing?"
> "Grandma," in exasperation, "you just open your eyes!"

There are, of course, streams and ponds for the cattle that roam these grasslands where once only bison lived. But what makes this land unique is the miles and miles of grasslands. You can turn in a circle and see from horizon to horizon: one big blue vault over tall grass. The key is, you have to be able to look at "nothing" before you can see anything. And there is so much to see.

I have learned to "see" Kansas by removing from my mind images of forests, seas, and mountains. They have no place here. People from the coasts can long for the comfort of those familiar sights, or they can clear them from their minds and experience prairie.

On some days the sky is clear. On other days, puffy clouds appear. Clouds that look like I could catch up with them at the top of the next hill, except that they don't wait for me. When the skies are leaden, sometimes I can see rain march across the prairie toward me. On certain days, especially in May, the sky menaces with the threat of tornadoes, and in this huge theater, there are times when I can see a number of black tails whip down out of the clouds and pull up again.

But no matter the weather, the prairie seems to confront me with my own mortality. Beyond its stark beauty, I can be vulnerable to oppressive heat, bitter cold, drought, rain, tornado, winter wind or summer wind, and my own fears of things I do not understand—like death.

June 20

"Your Mother is dying."

The doctor tells us that Mother is dying, but he shrugs his shoulders when we ask him the inevitable question, "When?" "Tomorrow or three months" is his answer.

It began about six years ago, when Mother became short of breath and lightheaded. Then one day while riding her bicycle in the little town of Hope, she fainted and fell into the ditch. Finally, after a year, she was diagnosed as having mitral valve prolapse, and with the advice of her doctor and at the urging of several of her children, she had open-heart surgery in Wichita. She was a good candidate for surgery because the rest of her body was in good condition, but since she was older, the physicians decided to use living tissue (pig) valves instead of artificial ones to replace her worn-out valves.

After Mother had the surgery and was recuperating at our home on Park Place, she picked up a book that had just come, called *Whole Body Healing*, and in it she read that the living tissue valves would last approximately five years. She didn't say anything to us, just laid the book aside. I think she was wondering why she had gone through all that pain for a five-year extension to such a full life. Like her, until I saw the book, I did not know the time-line for the living tissue valves was so short. The doctors had not discussed with her or with the family that there was a choice. Nor what the consequences of the choice they made for her would be. It seemed as if a cruel hoax had been perpetrated on her.

During the years following that surgery, she frequently said she would never go through that again.

Now, the replaced valves have worn out. They have caused stress on her heart. It, too, is dying.

June 23

Her Time to Die

I have spent the past three days at the hospital, sleeping at night in a chair in Mother's room. The fluid was drained from around her heart, and she has been stabilized with drugs. Now I begin the hundred-mile journey home to get some rest. It is evening and the sky is ablaze with the setting sun. Amid the brilliance, there is a rift in the clouds, and streaks of light connect the earth. Out of my past come the words of an old hymn . . . "Heaven came down and glory filled my soul." I begin to sing there under the open sky with its huge pink-tinged clouds. And I remember that once there was a little girl named Carol whose mother Alice so loved the sunset that she often went west beyond the apricot grove into the pasture to watch those brief moments before dark. I can still see her standing in the glow of the setting sun. That same sun now comforts me and fills my soul with the certainty that death is part of life.

I think back to the months before her open-heart surgery, after the doctor diagnosed the mitral valve prolapse. The leak in her heart caused her to panic when she was alone. Her fear often subsided when we were there because she focused on us. The operation helped lessen her panic, but within the last year, as the replacement valves wore out, the panic returned. For the first time in her life, our Mother, who had always put others before herself, had begun to be self-centered. It was hard to see her that way. But she had been alone for long periods of time, having what I now know as increasing periods of agitation caused by the leakage in her heart. I'm not sure that anyone took time to explain to her that her panic was common to people with this problem. I think she never asked, just assuming it was something she had to get through, the way she had to get through life. Soon she won't need any answers. The anger and frustration at things no longer important to her threaten to overwhelm me. I purposely concentrate on the clouds.

This is my Mother's land and my Mother's sunset and my Mother's God. I am a traveler here, and I am watching and listening and wondering and accepting all that comes to me. This will be my last gift to my Mother. I am going with her as far as I can on this journey.

Undated

"Mom, do you know what you've just signed?"

We are all gathered in the room, six family members and three nurses sent in from the administrative offices. They have some papers for Mother to sign, and since she is too weak to sign her name, they are here to witness her mark. Helen props her up and holds her hand. Mother is worn out and everyone is quiet as she falls back against the bed. Suddenly my brother, John, calls out, "Mom, Mom, do you know what you've just signed?" Mother looks perplexed and John announces emphatically, "You've just joined the army!" Amid hoots of laughter, I see Mother's grin and in her eyes a flicker of appreciation. This use of humor as a defense against stark truth is a mark of a true Kansan. And no one was better at it than our Mother.

The first few generations of Kansans, descendants of the plains settlers, were good at enduring trouble with laughter. And in the Kansas of the 1800s there was much disaster to overcome. To my knowledge, the first person to identify this Kansas humor was Carl Becker, writing in the 1920s. He said Kansans employ humor as a defense against misfortune. A current writer, Randy Brown of Wichita, adds that Kansans are not about to allow good times to stand in the way of their discontent.

Carl Becker described the problems of a farmer during a rainy Kansas spring. The wheat was probably ruined and no corn had yet been planted. The farmer's profits were wiped out, but he looked at the murky sky, sniffed the damp air, and remarked, "Well, it looks like rain. We may save that crop yet." "Yes", his neighbor replied, "but it will have to come soon, or it won't do any good."

Becker goes on to tell how during the grasshopper invasion, when grasshoppers were six inches deep in the street, the editor of a Kansas paper wrote this single line: "A grasshopper was seen on the court-house steps this morning." And more recently my brother John, talking to a visitor from England who had only been in the States for three days, said with mock seriousness, "It's remarkable how good you are with the language, no longer than you've been here."

Kansas humor comes from a long line of people who remember what it was to face disaster after disaster, people who "stuck it out" and, according to Becker, endured all Kansas had to inflict by way of natural disasters—drought, grasshopper invasions, and tornadoes. They stayed, they kept the faith, and with their endurance came a certain pride in their efforts, a feeling of superiority that came from a victory they almost didn't win.

Becker says that many Kansas pioneers felt endurance was its own reward, since there were no worse worlds to conquer. A Kansan doesn't endure with a martyr's air, Becker goes on to explain, but rather, transforms a disaster into a minor annoyance by making a joke of it.

Kansas humor is handed down from generation to generation. You hear it first as a child, begin to employ it as an adult, and have it mastered by old age. Uncle Orville was particularly good at it, as was my Grandfather John. My Father's unique storytelling was enhanced by it. For my brother, my sister, and me, humor is often a communal sort of thing, where we sit around bantering—and it can go on forever—until one of us comes up with a line that breaks us up. We all know it is coming, we just don't know which one of us will get there first!

Or it can be the result of one person's dry comments. That is more my Mother's style, and it is often unexpected.

Today, when John told her that with the signing of the hospital papers she had joined the army, our Mother lay there, looking death in the face and laughing.

June 24

> Donavon says, "The owl wants to know 'who,' and the
> mourning dove laments 'why.'"

Highway 4 stretches before me as I run the doglegs through
Latimer, White City, Dwight, and Alta Vista toward Topeka.
Grasses flow across the horizon. Sun and wind and grass and
me, alone and sleepy. I pull onto an intersecting dirt road and
stop. I am reasonably sure there will be no traffic, but I pull
way over to the side, open the windows, lie back, and go to
sleep with the sun warm on my face.

The prairie, under the intense light of a sky-span from horizon to horizon, is the only place I have ever felt so totally
open. There is no place to hide. No music, no intrusions,
no other people . . . only the wind moving the grass.

I wake twenty minutes later to the song of Mother's favorite
bird, the meadowlark. As usual, I can hear it but I can't see
it. It's easy to miss prairie birds. The meadowlark nests in the
grasses along the road and sits on fences to warble the cheerful song known to all tall-grass people. At night owls call.
Often, in the silence of the grasslands, great migrations
of waterfowl pass overhead so far away that you cannot hear
their call as they fly this stretch of the open corridor from
Canada to eastern Mexico.

Many prairie birds leave in the winter, but the ones that stay, like the prairie chicken, with its staccato dance and booming voice, and the quail, pull back into the shrubs along the waterways. Smaller birds roost in cedar trees, and when they fly, join together in a large flock of many different tiny birds. Crows also fly in huge flocks to roost in the cities of Kansas at night and fly out to feed on the croplands during the day. In the winter, raptors rule the wide expanse of grass.

Still sleepy, still listening, at last I hear the musical wood-flute tone of the mourning dove floating across the prairie. "Why, oh why . . . why,why,why,why?"

As I start the car, I try to imagine how far I've come. I must be in Wabaunsee County. I smile, thinking about my recent conversation with a friend who observed, "Rural Kansans always say they are from Dickinson County, or Greenwood County, or Saline County, or whatever county it is they hail from." She was right. We don't say, "I live at RR2 Hillsboro." We say, "I'm from Marion County." If they have farm roots, even longtime Wichitans say they live in Sedgwick County, even though they live in the largest city in Kansas. Perhaps this method of identifying where we live has to do with pre-serving a sense of community in a state with 105 counties.

The sun is low in the sky. The prevailing grass around me is a tall prairie grass known as bluestem. Further west beyond the Flint Hills grows a mid-level grass called grama, and in western Kansas, what you'll find most often is buffalo grass, a short grass. As I drive, the bluestem prairie falls behind me and farmland begins to appear.

The fields along this narrow road are planted to crops, but just outside the fences grows the tall grass. Even in the fall, when the fields are plowed and the ground is dark and rich, the grasses will be there at the edge of the fields. They wait with their companion sunflowers. If the farmer falls lax just a couple of years, the grass will begin an inward journey, moving to reclaim the land. Some tall grasses have existed almost one hundred years just outside the Osage orange fence posts with their rusted strands of wire. Alone and forever vigilant.

I pass Eskridge and go north through Keene, then east through Dover, and finally reach Topeka. Loneliness hangs heavy on me as I walk from the garage to the house. The rosy sky is fading fast, but in the window I see Donavon reading, unaware I am home. Lamplight spills across the room and out the window. The familiar pieces of my life are in there, with my husband. I reach for the doorknob. Behind me, perched high on a wire, a mourning dove laments, "Why, oh why . . . why,why,why,why?"

June 26

"Hi Mother! Did you have a good sleep last night?"
"I didn't stay awake to find out."

Mother seems content in the hospital. She did not want to live alone after a broken hip in January, nor did she want to be a burden to her children. She had been living with Helen these last few months and was happy there, but in the hospital, she feels that she no longer will suffer from anxiety and panic. She believes she will get help.

The kind of help she wants comes as a surprise to us. After the last surgery, she had told all of us she never wanted to go through surgery again. Now Helen and I meet with the doctor in his office, finding out what Mother's options might be. He says a heart specialist could examine her to determine if she could have further surgery. But since Mother has repeatedly said she does not want further surgery, the heart specialist should not be asked to make a trip here. We agree. We go back to her room and she asks, "What did the doctor say?" We discuss the options. Death or further surgery if the heart is not too damaged. In about forty-five seconds she decides. With a sigh she says, "I guess we'd better go with the surgery." Astonished, I say, "All right, I will tell the doctor." When we go back to his office, it is closed, so I leave a note under his door.

It is a false hope. Within a few days we get word the heart specialist has determined from talking with Mother's doctor and reviewing her record that she is not a good candidate for surgery and would die during an operation. Now we have to tell her it is too late. She listens quietly. From this point on, we will simply wait.

It is quiet in Mother's room. Several days ago, a cricket made its way into the room and serenaded us. Yesterday the exterminator came to spray around the walls and in the halls. Last night our lone cricket chirped and then there was no more noise. Mother and I had enjoyed the cricket. It reminded us of summer nights across Kansas.

On the farm, with windows open, we could hear crickets tuning up, katydids trying to outdo the crickets' chorus, coyotes on some far-off ridge joining in around dawn, a restlessness in the hen house, a listening on the prairie.

Now, sitting in this quiet, sterile room, I wish for the sound of the cricket.

19

It is getting dark. I tell Mother I am going back to Topeka, and then I ask if she wants me to leave the lights on or off. She says, "Leave that light on please." I look at the place where she motioned. There is no light there, only the television. I go to the door and switch on the lights. "No," she quickly says, "that one." Again, she points to the television. I finally understand. The nursing staff often leaves the television on for her, giving her visual company with no sound. I feel grateful to them for all their little kindnesses.

I go home in the sunset again. The clouds look as if they will explode with their magnificent color. On the opposite side of the sunset, clouds pick up a hint of mauve to create a fantastic skyscape. My world is really not empty. It is full of earth and sky and grass. And I have a rightful insignificant place here.

Tonight on the prairie, as with every time I go back and forth between the hospital and home, I am aware I am just one small speck in the midst of the grasslands. But now there is a new awareness. This day I know what I am—an almost unseeable part of the whole. In amazement I realize I have never really been in control of most of the things in my life. Those things I do control are quite insignificant. I cannot take my Mother's dying and make her well. I cannot fix it this time. How unbelievably comforting it is to be only one small part of this vast land and how safe to be a part of this mysterious happening that I don't have to control.

June 27

I am stumped. The poem eludes me. I begin again and look toward my brother. John shrugs. Mother, whom I had believed asleep, murmurs. We stoop to hear. Her voice gets stronger as she recites the poem from beginning to end.

We grew up listening to Mother rhyme her way through pans full of dishes, washerloads of clothes, and baskets full of ironing. Canning was always accompanied by poetry.

How many times have I seen my Mother stop stirring apple butter on the stove and say, "Oh, there was a poem in the *Ladies Home Journal* . . . ," quote it halfway through and then . . . "Oops!" go back to stirring before the apple butter burned to the pan. The poetry may have been doggerel, but it was also mental gymnastics when the body was doing something boring.

As a child, I hated going to get the mail because it was a quarter-mile walk down our lane to the mailbox. To an impetuous little girl, that quarter-mile was a long way. So Mother would entice me with a variation on "Carrie, Carrie, get the mail / In a basket or in a pail / Plenty of sunshine and no hail / Please go out and get the mail!" When I fell and skinned my knee, Mother would rhyme while she applied iodine: "Carrie, Carrie, little Carrie / Has a knee that isn't hairy. / If she looked more like Burt, / Her knee just would not get so hurt!"

I don't know how far back it began. But my grandmother Clara Robinson and her sisters had access to the library of their father, "Squire" Robinson, in Hope. Like many prairie women, they read and copied poetry in the days before radio or television waves were beamed across the prairie. They would find a passage they particularly liked, write it out in flowing cursive, and send it to their friends or family who, of course, would put it in a scrapbook.

Paper was not plentiful, and they would often copy poetry on the back of "used" pages. There were two reasons for copying it: first, it was a pleasure to see it in their own hand-writing, and second, it was then committed to memory. I have an old leatherbound ledger from the creamery in Hope in which the clerk listed the products and amounts brought in from the neighboring farmers, and which, when it was discarded, ended up in my Grandmother's possession. Her intent, of course, was to use the pages that were not filled. So, in the back of this ledger, following the entries of eggs, butter, cream, and milk, are poems—poems in Grandma's then strong handwriting and poems in the beginning scrawl of my Mother at age seven.

For these women of the prairie, it was only a short leap from copying poetry in a scrapbook to making up their own. No one said it had to be good, but everyone was expected to participate. The message that came down was "it's okay to express oneself in poetry." Out on the prairie, far from the ways of their foremothers, far from the acknowledged culture of the eastern states, their own poetry became the marker for a culture in transition. They all did it, amazed that there were people who didn't dare to try.

Traveling the early dusk home through the Flint Hills, I now think about one of the first poems I wrote as a child. It was written during the crystal beauty of an icy winter day when our family was isolated on the farm, with no way in or out until the storm was over. From that day to this, I have written poetry. It is not good poetry, but it says what cannot be easily said in prose, and it is my inheritance from the women of my Grandmother's family. What a heritage!

Sh-h-h, listen carefully. Can you hear the slap, slap, slap of Mother's hands, kneading bread in a kitchen on a prairie farm south of Hope?

June 28

"Mother, does your head hurt?"
"Does my toe hurt?"
"It does? What else hurts?"
(Wryly) "A pain in the neck."

She wants me to quit asking how she is feeling. Our little
stoic Mother was taught as a child not to let others know
when she was hurting. Now that habit is beginning to create
a problem for her. When we try to obtain medication, the
nursing staff does not believe she is in pain.

Today we learn Mother's church in Hope finally has a minister after a time without. We think Mother is asleep, so Helen
and I wonder aloud when he'll come to the hospital. Her
eyes are still closed, but Mother says, "Tell him I'm going to
fire him if he doesn't come."

She seems agitated, so I caution her, "Mother you'd better
be careful or I'll sing to you." I hear a snicker and see a nurse
disappearing out the door. The male nurse still in her room
turns his head so I won't see him smile. They must have
heard me sing.

It has been still in the hospital room. Mother raises herself
and looks at us. Using Helen's nickname, she says, "You and
Honey lie down and rest." Memories wash over me. For the

past twenty years, whenever I visited her in Hope she would insist I lie down and rest before starting home. Now here we are in her hospital room, she is dying, and her concern is, as always, "You and Honey lie down and rest." Sometimes she will say, "We're all tired. We all need to rest," trying to include us in her agenda. "Okay, Mama," Helen says, "we are going to sleep. You sleep, too." And Mother closes her eyes.

So many friends and relatives have come to see Mother. Her niece Bernadell often stops by after work. Today, her cousin Opal tells Helen and me about the Model T that Mother and her sister Edna drove to teach school. Opal says, "With Edna, it was a smooth ride, with Alice it was wild." I look at Mother. Her eyes are closed. She pretends to be asleep but I don't let her get by with it. "Oh Mother, you drove like Helen does!" Her lips suppress a smile. Helen and I grin at each other.

It is time to go. I write out our phone numbers again to leave at the nurses' desk. I know they already have them, but I feel better doing it. I tell Mother I'm going back to Topeka. She nods a weak little nod. I bend over, give her a kiss, and in a stage whisper I say, "I'm so sorry to have to leave you alone with Helen." She responds in the same old way, "Oh, I believe I'll survive."

She hears us both laugh. That is what she was after. "Okay, Mother, I'll be back when you need me . . . or when I need you." She smiles.

June 29

"Hi, Mother. I see you have some more cards."
"Well, should we read them or send them back?"

Helen has taped Mother's cards to the wall. I smile when I
see them because I know our brother, John, will tease her
about them. He'll say, "Helen's been at work again. Didn't
she get enough of this in grade school?" Mother will lie in
bed and enjoy the arguing and pretend she doesn't hear.

The cards are not coming as often as they did at first. Helen
says she never knew before how much the family depends on
cards. I'm sure that it is difficult for Mother's friends and relatives to select cards to send her. It is difficult for me. Mother
loved cards. They were her method of communication. She
sent cards to everyone for every reason she could think of
and some just because. She sent cards to family, neighbors,
acquaintances of decades before, and even surviving spouses
of people she once knew and loved.

A month ago I bought Mother a card with aspens on it
because she always loved leaves. She is the reason I love fall.
Now I pause at card counters and turn away. What is there
to say that hasn't been said? What in all these stacks of cards
will bring her comfort? They all want her to get well and go
home. Yesterday I found one that had a cuddly bear on it and

a verse that said, "I want to put my arms around you and hold you forever." It was perfect, and I had to fight back tears as I took it to the counter and paid for it.

Tonight, on the road going home, I think of the messages I read today in Mother's room, each unique to the sender. I hold the steering wheel with my left hand, and because I have forgotten my tape recorder, lean to the passenger side and scribble on the side of a grocery sack, "now in this lonesome room, sometime between dawn and noon, her children hear from day to day, a voice she touched along her way."

At home, I carry in the sack, glance at the lines, and remembering the messages at Mother's bedside, open up my laptop computer to write "Song of the Get Well Cards."

Please get well! Please get well!
They line the walls and make a shell.
The new ones lie upon the table
Perhaps she'll open them when she's able?

Now in this lonesome room
Midway between dawn and noon
Her children hear from day to day
A voice she touched along the way.

"Dear Aunt Alice, we went to the volleyball game last night, we missed you and we are praying for you . . ." "Dear Grandma, the picture on the front of this card reminds me of you reading to me . . ." "Dear Great-grandmother, I remember your quiet smile and I miss the smells of your kitchen and your snickerdoodles . . ." "My dear sister, we shared so many special times and it brings me happiness to think of them . . ." "Dear Alice, the Lord is seeing to every detail that concerns you but at church and sunday school, we miss you . . ." "Dear Cousin, I am thinking of you and remembering the fun times, they were so long ago but I could never forget . . ." "Dear Grandma, your faith in God has helped me so much this past year, you are a remarkable woman and special to me . . ." "Dear Teacher, you were my favorite teacher, so kind and so funny, I learned so much and you were the best . . ." "Dear Friend, we had such good times and you helped me, too. I am sorry you are sick, please come back soon . . ."

Please get well! Please get well!
They line the walls and make a shell
Around the one who's lying there
Who cannot read, who cannot care.

Here in her history's afterglow
The passing of this gentle soul
Has brought forth those who loved her long
Who by their cards, now sing her song.

SILENCE

They say there is a place of silence, in the chapel in the city.

I tried it once. Sitting in a honey-pine pew, with red carpet on the kneeling board, seeing sunlight filtering through colored panes of glass, I waited, all alone, for silence.

I heard a constant drone of cars streaming by, trucks pulling upgrade a mile away, air conditioners wheezing and whistling, an occasional shout breaking the murmur of people's voices.

Today on the prairie, I knew silence. It was around and over and through me. It flowed over the rises and breaks. It rushed across the flint and the seed and pressed upon me until I felt as if I had grown like an Atlas of the grasslands, flinging wide my arms to touch the sky, holding up all my silence.

A raptor's wings beat the air. A straight dive, a shrill cry in the quivering grass. Hawk now rising, heavy burden dragging. Flying higher and higher, to reach some prairie haunt to fill its body . . . like silence fills my soul.

ON THE
PRE-AGRARIAN
PRAIRIE

Second Scene

Now the sun has its way. There is no place to hide. Sleep after sleep, sun upon sun, the temperature exceeds one hundred degrees. Hot days blend into warm nights. Tall grasses sag toward the ground, dying in the scorch of sun, while grass-hoppers and crickets search around roots with ever-weakening chirps. Huge cracks zigzag in uncertain patterns across the plain.

Hawks find banquets spread below them. Prairie dogs remain in their burrows, sucking moisture from grass they have stored under the sod. Heat pulses into the cooler earth, while above, in lazy circles, eagles float.

Bison, with bushy, black-brown fur crackling in the sun, plod distractedly from one dried-up water hole to the next. The herd moves faster and faster in search of water while the old and sick, unable to keep up, fall underneath the rays of the sun and cook where they lie. Deer have long since gone into the west. From horizon to horizon, there is not a single cloud. There is only the sun and heat and silence.

FROM THE DIARY
IN JULY

July 2

"Soli Deo Gloria"

I arrive at the hospital early. I'm going to spend some time with Mother and then head to central Kansas. Uncle Sam, one of our Father's younger brothers, died last week and today is his funeral. We told Mother about his death and she listened. We knew she understood but she is dealing with her own death now.

She has begun to pray almost continually. "Help me Father, help me to do what's right. I pray in Jesus' name. Amen. Help me Father, help me to do what's right. I pray in Jesus' name. Amen. Help . . ." Nurses interrupt her, and I noticed last week it has become very uncomfortable for Helen. She will call "Mother, Mother!" just to stop the incessant praying. I think Mother does not know she prays constantly. I think her praying is like a mantra and it helps comfort her.

Today, I ask her if she wants me to pray and she nods. I wonder what will comfort her, and then I just pray what is in my mind. "Our Father who art in heaven, take care of your servant Alice. We don't mean to tell you what to do, just ask you to watch over her and then in your good time take her home to be with you. She has suffered so much. We thank you for her love so great all these years. Your love is the only love greater than hers for us. Be with her now. In Jesus' name, amen." She whispers, "Amen."

I leave the hospital to join my brother, John, and my sister, Helen, at the funeral in Hutchinson. I have underestimated the travel time, and so I cut across the country on an unknown road through farmland and ripe wheat. Wheat was the main source of income on my childhood farm. We lived from one harvest to another, and our income depended on the weather. If the wheat harvest was rained out or hailed out, we knew the coming year would be lean. But there would always be another year, another harvest. How many days have I stood under a stormy Kansas sky watching the thin wheat stems with their full heads flowing into a massive, undulating yellow sea. Wishing, as little children wish, I could put an umbrella over the field or a bucket under the hail and with my arms outstretched, hold back the wind. Now I find myself remembering those farmers of my youth, who, like my Father, knew they could not change the weather. They learned to live with the land, planting what the ground would accept, avoiding crops unsuited for Kansas, crops that depleted their water sources. They understood and accepted the limitations of weather and land.

I arrive at the church and slip into the pew with just minutes to spare. I glance back at John and Helen, who look relieved to see me. The good thing about my habitual tardiness is no one ever really expects to see me until I'm there. Mother was the one exception. She always expected me to be on time. But the others have been overheard to say "Carol will be late to her own funeral!" I have commissioned my niece, Robin, to be sure I don't disappoint them when that day arrives.

The service is comforting, and I am pleased to find Uncle Sam was well respected in his community. It feels right to be with everyone at the family dinner afterward. But in the back of my mind is the knowledge I never told Uncle Sam how proud I was to be his niece. I wish I had told him.

Although Mother's parents, John and Clara Anderson, were Swedish-English, my Father's parents, George and Eva Brunner, were German. Their ancestors, at the request of the Russian leader, Catherine the Great (also German), settled the Volga region of Russia. Many of her people moved to that uncared-for land, taming and farming it. In exchange, they were free to live in villages they created, worship the way they wanted, speak their own language, and educate their children as Germans. Catherine's promises lasted more than a century, but by the time George and Eva were married, the political climate had changed, and these Germans who had made the Volga area prosperous were now threatened with losing their German identity.

The farmland the Brunners had made into a profitable horse raising business was taken by the government. Two years after George Brunner married Eva Beisel, they left Saratof, Russia, and came to the New World with their baby, Henry, who learned to walk on board the ship. Entering through Ellis Island, they crossed America and arrived in Hope, Kansas, on April 22, 1892, George's twentieth birthday.

By 1898 they had purchased the farm two miles north of Ramona that is still called "the Home Place." Thirteen children were born to these hardy immigrants, my Father, Daniel, being the eighth child. I often thought it was curious that my Father, who had been born on U.S. soil, could not speak English until he went to school and then was required to speak German at home. Not until I was grown and heard the story of the Germans from Russia did I realize how deeply ingrained in the members of this family was the desire to keep their heritage alive. That is why they came here and that is how they lived for a generation.

In many German settlements across Kansas, farming was enhanced because of these hardworking settlers, who only wanted a place in which to work and raise their children and worship as they had in the Old Country.

Our family grew, and now there are many of us in the United States who trace our heritage to George and Eva. In a family history written by Rev. Gene Hicks is this tribute: "Descendants of these brave and God-fearing people stand in awe of the many accomplishments and progress shown by this stalwart generation. Without medical aid and help, without the assistance, often time, of doctors, children were born and reared to adulthood. Soli Deo Gloria!"

I return to the hospital, thinking about the religious and social differences of my parents' backgrounds, wondering if they knew the depths of each other's history and just why they were the way they were. But we are beyond that now.

In the evening I come out of the hospital into the lingering heat of the summer sun. Getting into my car, I begin the long trip back. Just for a moment I let down and cry. I cry for the Uncle I didn't know very well, and then for myself and what I am about to face, and I cry for my Mother because it now no longer matters. There is something terribly final when life no longer matters.

I am aware the trip will be long, but soon I am caught up in the healing depth of it, the vast sky and the endless rolling prairie. Once again, I accept the feeling of total aloneness. And I begin to see . . . the grass changing hue from one hill to the next. And now there are shadows on the hills. Darkness is coming.

July 3

> The prairie comes to color in the fall when tall
> grasses bloom, when sumac is deep red, and when
> fog lies heavy in low areas. Then do the shadowed
> hills look like purple glaciers.

I have driven far and braved deep ruts to get here. The road
is no longer, it ends in pasture. There is no sound now except
for the humming of a bee. A jet plane is making a vapor trail
across the sky. I kneel down and look deep into the grass.

You have to do that to see the hundreds of different kinds of
grasses that make up what we call grassland but which is literally a community of plants. Each species contributes to the
amazingly complex prairie. All are living in a fragile ecology
of dirt about six inches deep.

There is not just one color, but tiny dots of many colors
like lithographs or offset printing. Donavon says if you really
want to see the prairie, go look at a Birger Sandzén landscape. Your first reaction will be, "Prairie doesn't look like
that." But one day you'll look at the prairie and the light will
be just right and you will say, "Well, yes it does!" Umbers,
ochers, siennas, greens, and reds are blended, even in the
dead of winter. And in the winter, you don't see the green
until you get right up to it and peer down into it. If the green

weren't there, the color of the hills would be different. In fact, if any color were missing, the prairie would not be the same.

I sit back in the grass and think of this bluestem, which can rise over six feet high when it blooms. Kansas folklore tells of children getting lost and adults standing in the stirrups of their horses to see over the grass.

It is best to travel of a morning or evening, because of the angle that the light hits the hills when the sun is low. When you look south into the rolling prairie, the hills are lighted on one side and shadowed on the other. This light shining on the varieties of color provides a magenta effect to the grass that creates our "purple" hills. (We Kansans call them "hills" but they are actually rolling prairie.)

Today, the color does not matter. I came to fill my soul with silence. I am ready to go home.

July 6

Anders' Son

I am on the road to see Mother, this time heading southeast
from Abilene under huge puffy white clouds so low that
surely if I open the window I can reach up and touch them. I
laugh at myself, remembering childhood days playing games
with the clouds. Going out to get the mail and coming back
down the lane, stopping to let my bare feet snuggle down in
the soft fine dirt . . . a shadow runs across the ground. I look
up. Another one. Now I wait with a gleam in my eye. Here
comes a big one! I let it catch up and race it down the long
lane, trying to stay in its shadow. I am always outdistanced
by my adversarial cloud, and I stand panting in the sunlight
once more, watching the mosaic on the fields of my youth.

I snap out of my reverie and think about Mother, feeling that
I have neglected her a little. For the last three days we have
been at a camp on the Smoky Hill River with my Anderson/
Robinson cousins, some of whom have come from as far
away as Florida and Minnesota. Tom Anderson and I planned
this reunion before Mother was hospitalized. At the time we
organized it—our Uncle Orville had died and we were tired
of meeting only at funerals.

So we had this one-time reunion, and the only thing that
spoiled it was that it came too late for Mother. Several aunts

and cousins left the reunion from time to time and went to the hospital to visit her. They returned quiet.

Oh how she would have enjoyed it! A major part of our reunion was spent on genealogy. A highlight came when Mother's cousin Jim Anderson showed a video of his trip to Sweden and the church where the Anderson family records were stored. Our first known Anderson ancestor was Gabriel Larrson, whose son was Anders Gabrielson. Anders' son was called Swen Anderson.

In 1857, Swen, his wife Majastina, and their family sailed to America and settled in New Sweden, Iowa. One son of this family was Carl, who was two years old when they left Sweden. The ship's officer wrote Charles instead of Carl in the passenger list, and so the name he took in America was Charles Anderson. From that time on, following English custom, the family name was Anderson. According to Joe Brewer's history, Charles left home to join the Union army, serving in Company E, the 45th Iowa Infantry. After the Civil War he came to Shawnee County, Kansas, and in 1870 married Mary Falen. They lived near Wakarusa for nine years and then came across the Flint Hills to homestead west of Hope, Kansas. His son John was my Mother's father.

I have fond memories of my grandparents' farm. Dominating the farmyard was a big red barn and, in the workshop, a forge built by Charles. The forge was fed by a coal fire blown by a huge six-foot wood and leather bellows that hung from the rafters. East of the house was the washhouse, with its wood stove and kettles. There my Grandmother and her mother washed the clothes.

Now I sit by Mother's side, trying to tell her of the past three days. She is weak and pale. She has been repeating over and over . . . "I hope, I pray. I hope, I love." It is a precious mantra and I hate to interrupt, but I have something to say I know she will want to hear. She had been so proud of her father and will want to know all I have learned about her people. "Mother," I say, "just listen to this!" She smiles a little. I read from my notes, excitedly telling her about Anders' son, Swen. If they had stayed in Sweden for one more generation, I tell her, we'd be Swensons, not Andersons! I glance toward the bed. She has fallen asleep.

July 8

I close my eyes to see myself when I was five. There are tree limbs around me on all sides, sweeping the ground, the walls of my secret room. Discarded dishes sit in the crook of a tree, my doll lies on a cedar bed. Helen crawls in. "Don't tell John we're here," she whispers. I can hear him calling in the distance.

Today, sitting comfortably in my Adirondack chair on the patio back of my Topeka home, I watch squirrels beg for sunflower seeds. I'm thinking about the tour I organized for my cousins when they were home several days ago. We started at the Anderson farm on Highway 4 west of Hope. The house was falling in, but the big red barn, now in need of paint, still stood. The lane was almost impassable, and grasses had reclaimed the yard where Grandmother used to plant flowers. We drove five miles south of Hope, where, east of the Schimming farm and north of Huenquenet Cave, my parents' farm used to be. There is nothing left but a windmill and stock tank. Our next stop, one mile south of my parents' farm and half a mile west of Lauren Brunner's prosperous ranch, was at Aunt Edna's farm where the buildings are now dying in the grass. We ended our tour three miles east of Hope at the Robinson homestead, still a working farm.

Along the way, I heard one of my eastern cousins murmur something about "losers." I was amazed. These abandoned farm sites are important pieces of our history. They represent a way of life our ancestors developed that withstood grass-hopper plagues, dust storms in the Dirty Thirties, and the Great Depression. Those small farms were the backbone of the nation until the 1950s. Then, only our cousins who diversified and bought large amounts of acreage survived. But from those first agrarians who broke the sod of Kansas, there is nothing left except abandoned farm sites, standing in mute testimony to what once was.

When I was a child, entire families were supported by quarter-section farms that grew up at the edge of the Flint Hills where the soil was deeper and more fertile. Behind our house was a windbreak (shelter belt). Windbreaks were planted across Kansas so the soil would never again blow away as it did in the 1930s, the inevitable aftermath of the first sod-breaking by the early settlers. The shelter belt on our farm was a unique blend of cedar and apricot trees. Besides preserving the soil and sheltering wild game, it protected our house from northern winds each winter, provided 120 quarts of fruit each summer, gave up a Christmas tree each December, and provided the best playhouse any child could ever want.

Of all the barns, granaries, henhouses, corrals, and milk sheds that supported the family enterprise, usually only the windmill and silos remain intact on abandoned farm sites. The windmills were perhaps the single most important part of the farms. My Father used to tell of a windmill repairman who would sleepwalk, climb a windmill, and repair it in his sleep. Daddy said no one was to wake him or he would fall, and the windmill repairman was important to the farm community.

Listening for wind changes was part of the rhythm of prairie life. The sounds of a creaking windmill lulled many a farm family to sleep, got many a farmer out of bed at night when the wind increased, and brought water above ground to sustain life. The windmill, one of the most familiar of all Kansas sights, has become so much a part of the prairiescape that it does not look like the intrusion it really is. Whether shiny and new and swinging in the wind, or broken and old and drooping toward the ground, the windmill will always symbolize survival to prairie people.

July 9

Three Roads to Hope

As I sip my first cup of coffee this morning, I ponder which way I will take to get to the hospital. By the third cup, I know I will take Kansas Highway 4. It is my favorite of the three ways to go from Topeka, in the oak-hickory forest area of Kansas, to Hope, on the western edge of the bluestem prairie.

Topeka is in northeastern Kansas, the home of the native Kansa who lived in permanent villages and farmed along the waterways on the fringe of the prairie. During the hunting season they moved out onto the prairie, lived in portable bison-hide tepees, and followed the great herds of bison that roamed the grasslands during warm months. When Europeans began to search for new places to live in the heart of America, many arrived at this jumping-off place in northeastern Kansas, where some of the more famous trails began. The Oregon Trail and the Leavenworth Pikes Peak Express Stage Line headed west from here in prestatehood days.

I often begin my trip to Hope on Interstate 70. Soon after leaving the colorful treed hills of Shawnee County, I am on the prairie where the sky meets the grass with nothing in between. Westward I speed through the rolling hills of Wabaunsee County on a smooth four-lane highway.

Frequent "flyers" know the flashing of oncoming car lights are sympathetic drivers letting you know a highway patrol car sits just over the hill.

In some places the rolling prairie hills are so steep that cuts have been made through them. Within those cuts, I am shielded from wind but not for long. The wind catches me as I emerge from the cut and pushes at my car like a petulant child against its mother's leg.

Now I pass the Konza experimental plots, which belong to Kansas State University (the first land-grant college), located north of me in Manhattan. Reaching Geary County and topping a rise, I see Fort Riley, the "Big Red One," spread across the valley below. As I drop down the hill, World War II cannons perch high above me, while below on level plain, helicopters and HumVee's stand at parade rest amid the buildings of the fort. Around a bend and west again, I reach the junction where the Republican and Smoky Hill rivers merge to form the Kaw River. The city there is appropriately called Junction City. I turn south on Highway 77, climb out of the valley, and cross the rise and fall of the west-to-east ripples of the grassy prairie sea. As I reach Morris County, the land levels out, and wheat fields, pastures, and barnyards prevail. I follow the Morris/Dickinson county line to one mile north of Herington where I take Kansas Highway 4 nine miles west until it curves into Hope.

Another road to Hope leaves Topeka via the Kansas Turnpike, angling southwest from Shawnee County thirty miles through Osage and Lyon counties to the bison range of many years ago. Nowhere is it easier to imagine great herds of those shaggy beasts thundering over a hill than when I travel the lonesome stretches of the Kansas Turnpike. Leaving the turnpike at the Admire exit, I travel west through Lyon and Morris counties on U.S. 56, intersected by solitary lanes. Above the undulating prairie, raptors soar looking for their next meal. I cross the Neosho River and reach Council Grove, a historic town of early settlers where native people once held council and signed honorless treaties with the U.S. government. Two routes parallel this way. The Kaw trail was used by the Kansa Indians as a trading trail many years before Europeans came. The Santa Fe Trail originated at Westport in Kansas City and was traveled by pioneers to points southwest. At random sites along the Santa Fe Trail, ruts from the wheels of westward-moving wagons remain. Leaving Council Grove, I head west across farmland. South of me is Diamond Springs, the westernmost place in Kansas to be raided by proslavery forces during the days of "bleeding Kansas." Soon I reach Herington and from there, Hope.

But today I have chosen Highway 4, which was once a major Kansas road connecting the small towns across central Kansas with the capital city, Topeka. Although it was the first paved road in Kansas, it is now forsaken for the convenience of more modern highways. But Highway 4, as any old-timer knows, is the best way to see central Kansas. I leave Shawnee County, drive the solitary hills of Wabaunsee, through the turns and over narrow bridges, between the rock fences and up over the skyline, then down across Morris County into Dickinson. It is still very easy to lose myself in the Flint Hills in Wabaunsee County, one of my favorite places to view the grassy hills. I don't head out there if I am low on gas or if the weather is uncertain. Our son Daniel once got caught in a sudden snowstorm in nearby Chase County. After his car ran out of gas, he burned some of his school notebooks in the back of his station wagon in order to keep warm until the next morning when a truck came through. At least that's what he told his professor.

On days when time is important, I take I-70, sometimes alternating with the Kansas Turnpike. On days like today, when I want to be soothed by the purple hills, I take Highway 4, the winding, twisting pathway of my grandparents.

July 13

I say to Mother, "Today is our 34th wedding anniversary.
Donavon said he'd keep me another 34 years. That's 68.
What do you think about that?" She says, matter-of-factly,
"He'd better be careful about his promises."

Donavon has a meeting to attend in Salina, one of the larger
cities on the northwestern side of the Flint Hills. So we make
a motel reservation for the night and plan to celebrate our
anniversary with a dinner after his meeting. It is a long,
straight road from Topeka to Salina and having someone
to talk with makes the time pass swiftly. When I am not the
driver, it is easy to lose perspective about where I am on the
grassy hills. I ride along and then glance up and see something I wasn't expecting, and I imagine how the early settlers
felt without any reference point.

Several years ago, Donavon and I, with Kasia and Dru, our
two oldest granddaughters, were driving west on I-70 when
suddenly we saw a herd of camels. Camels on the prairie?
They were so out of place that we immediately tried to think
of ways to make it fit into the things we know to be true.
Kasia said, "Maybe there's a zoo nearby." Dru asked if there
was a circus around. Don said, "I've driven farther west than
I thought!" Later I found that some cattle rancher was experi-
menting with camels because they eat scrubby plants cattle

don't eat. Camel grazing may cut down on the frequency with which the prairie must be burned.

Now I watch the new grass on either side of us. Most of this land along I-70 was burned off last spring. Fire is the reason for the survival of grasslands. It is a natural method of preventing the invasion of shrubs and trees, which bear their buds above ground and can be easily killed by fire. The nations of native people who lived on the prairie before the Europeans came knew there was a relationship between prairie life and fire, that grasses grew from charred meadows, and that trees did not belong there. Today's ranchers know that if regularly burned, grass will continue to survive year after year.

It is a unique experience to see the prairie burn at night. Fire burns up one hill and down the next; crawling along the ground in creeping tongues of color, moving in pitch black up and over and across and down, ever onward to where the backfire is set. Smoke frequently drifts across roads during the burning and there probably are alarmed strangers who stop a patrol car and report "a fire four miles back!"

I often think how the settlers must have dreaded prairie fires. If they had time, they could hitch horses to a plow and plow land in front of their homes, or set a backfire to create a space of charred earth over which no fire could leap. At such times, it would have been hard to think that prairie fires are necessary.

I like being a passenger, for I can concentrate on the prairie. Soon we reach Salina. I let Donavon out at his meeting and head southeast for Herington. When I arrive at the hospital, I find Mother weak and in pain. We talk for a while. She knows it is our anniversary and she jokes with me a little. I ask for some pain medication for her. The nurse says, "We can't give her anything. It might hasten her death." I am surprised. There are worse things than death, and suffering while dying is one of them. In the past week, I've come to realize that the hospital staff and I are not communicating well. Everything they are about is keeping Mother alive. What Mother and I are about is her dying. Her comfort while dying has become a second, lesser consideration to her caregivers when it should be the first.

In the evening I go back to Salina. Helen stays at the hospital because she is worried about Mother. After Donavon and I check our bags into the motel, we find a restaurant. Outside is a pay phone, so I call the hospital now in order to eat without wondering how things are. John answers and says they do not think she will live through the night. He talks to the nurse and she concurs. I tell him I will come back. I explain the situation to Don. He just smiles, and we go back to pick up our bags at the motel, where, of course, it is too late to get a refund. He doesn't say anything about our missed dinner. In the car he says, "Happy Anniversary, Carol." I am numb and quiet. Mother's impending death holds such impact over everything now. Everything else is insignificant.

We all spend the first part of the night at the hospital and Mother gets better. The nurse is apologetic that we left our celebration. We tell her she did the right thing to call us back, and at midnight we go to Hope to sleep a few hours at John's house.

July 14

"Hi Mother, how about a hug?"
"How about two of them?"

Today, after that bad night, she is cheerful when I first come in. She has a sweet smile on her face and she says, "I love you so much. I've loved you for a long, long time." "Not so long Mother, just fifty-three years."

Her prayer has changed. It is now "Help me Father, help me do what's right. Amen. Heavenly Father, forgive me and guide me. In Jesus' name, amen." One of the aides thinks something is bothering Mother, and Helen's husband, Tom, suggests she talk to a minister. "Listen," I say to them, " she is a humble person. She prays as she has always prayed." I have heard that prayer all my life.

Tom played a unique role in Mother's recent life. Home-bound because of his own heart problems, he prepared her meals during the past few months. They were good and healthful meals, and she was always grateful for them. Characteristically, though, she would not tell him when she didn't like what was set in front of her. Tom was amused to see her eat a bite, hide the next bite in her napkin, eat a bite, hide the next one, until her plate was clean. "Mom," he'd tease, "I'll put your napkin in the trash." "Oh no," she'd say, "I'll clean up after myself."

Today, Christy brings three-year-old Travis and baby Tyler to see their greatgrandma and Travis sings "Jesus Loves Me." Mother is oblivious to everyone else while she concentrates on Travis and his sweet little voice.

Kasia and Dru, daughters of our oldest son Lance, visited last week. Dru, at age eight, was the littlest Von Trapp in the play "Sound of Music" in Emporia, so the two girls sang selections from that musical. Mother listened intently to every word and every note. They sensed her interest and continued to sing until I grew tired. But she did not, and her greatgranddaughters rose to the occasion, standing shoulder to shoulder, singing their hearts out. I will never forget that sight.

None of the greatgrandkids need any thanks. They sense her appreciation and her intense interest.

Now Mother and I are alone. She says, "I just can't seem to get up for some reason or another." She is in pain and uncomfortable and still trying to be stoic. I say to her, "Mother, when Helen comes the two of us will raise you up and you'll feel better." She responds, "When Helen Rose comes, it's hard to tell what the three of us will do."

I think it is time to tell her something I have been wanting to say for a long time. She had two wishes for the end of her life: "If I can just be faithful unto death," and "If I can just keep my mind." She had worked in nursing homes, had seen a beloved older sister deteriorate until she didn't know those around her, and she had had an aunt who died at the Topeka State Hospital. The possibility of losing her mind bothered her so much that as she got older, she talked frequently to me about it.

Finally, three years ago, I said to her, "Mother, I promise you I will tell you if your mind gets bad." That seemed to console her. Today, I want to lay this fear to rest. I say to her, "Mother, you always told us you just wanted to keep your mind. . . . Well look, Mother, you did it!" She smiles at me.

Later, Helen and I put Mother in the wheelchair and leave for a cup of coffee. When we come back, Helen, smiling, bends over in front of her, making a circle of arms between them. Mother looks at her intently for several long seconds and then quietly says, "Love never fails."

July 16

Faithful unto death.

All of us are focusing on Mother's impending death, but she has been talking about it since I was a little child. She would say, "If I can just live until the kids are grown up . . . if I can just live until . . ." as though her death were imminent. At times I wondered if it was unhealthy for her to think about it so much.

I think that death to her is simply a part of living. She doesn't see it as a "bad thing." Certainly she never intended it as a threat to us. And in a way, it will come as no surprise to me when she does die. I am prepared.

Mother's faith is strong and her beliefs uncompromising. At times, this has created considerable dismay for her and more frequently for some of her family. It's not hard to imagine what an enormous effect her faith has on her living and her dying. Mother's religious persuasion is about as American as you can get; it was born in frontier Kentucky as theologians Campbell and Smith turned from traditional Protestant views to declare "no name but Christ, no creed but the Bible" and spawned a movement that was to become a major denomination. Only on the frontier, in the climate created there, could such a movement have succeeded.

Mother's religious inheritance goes back much further, however. According to research by my cousin, Phyllis Scofield, a direct ancestor of Mother's, John Robinson, graduated from Cambridge in the late 1500s and was involved in theological reform as the pastor of the Pilgrim church. After the imprisonment of some Pilgrim church members, 120 "souls" fled with pastor John on the Mayflower to Holland. They lived twelve years in Leiden while preparing to go to America. Finally the first of four boatloads set sail for the new land, arriving at Plymouth Rock in 1620. But Pastor John Robinson, at whose prompting "went forth the Pilgrim Fathers to settle New England in 1620," never made it to America. He died at the age of forty-nine and is buried in Leiden. His widow, Bridget White Robinson, and their son Issac came on the Handmaid, the fourth boat.

Today at the library I found a book containing letters from Robinson to the Pilgrims in America. At the end of some of his letters I see the words "If I can just remain faithful unto death." In amazement I wonder how many times have I heard my Mother say those words. Second only to her "I love you" was "If I can just remain faithful unto death."

When Donavon came home from work I read him the Robinson-Pilgrim letter and when I came to the phrase, he looked startled and said, "Why that's what Mom always said." Doni Marie concurred. A concern passed down for more than twelve generations has to be strong!

To understand her heritage is to understand Mother, and her heritage includes a man who, 350 years ago, encouraged his church to move to a new continent to find religious freedom. And it also includes more recent ancestors who embraced the independent Christian church, which on the American frontier declared its independence from religious hierarchy.

July 17

I won't be rained on when I die.

Today Donavon and I are sitting by her bed. She asks, "No one is listening to me, why am I here?" I sit silent, trying to say, and not knowing how to say, that she is dying. Don comes through for her by answering the question: "Mom, your heart is hurting and your kidneys are weak." "Oh yes," she says. We are quiet for a while and then she turns to me and says, "I thank God for His great love."

Later on, I try to get her to talk about death. I say to her, "Mother, do you know you are not going to get well?" "No, I didn't know that." It would be like her to say that just to see what I am going to say, but it could also be a response to the "get well" attitude of her medical attendants. So I say, "Your heart is wearing out, and when it does you will go home to be with Jesus and Daddy and your Poppa and Mama." I use the terms of endearment so familiar to her. She does not respond. By afternoon she rallies almost as if to tell me I am wrong.

On the way home, I think I am learning to keep my mouth shut, and I secretly sorrow for my Mother. What she always called "going home to be with Jesus" could have been, should have been, the highlight of her life. Instead, nobody wants to admit that Alice is dying.

One day, a minister from another church came in with his wife and child. He talked to Mother, said the usual comforting words, and gave a prayer that ended in a supplication for her good health. So I said to him, "Mother is going home to be with Jesus." He was visibly upset and left soon afterward. He had coped with death by encouraging her to think she was going to get up out of that bed and go home. That was the attitude of everyone around her. They didn't talk about dying, they talked about living.

Now I feel like the only naysayer. My belief in dignified dying surrounded by supportive people feels like a fanciful dream. I'm remembering her prayer this afternoon: "Heavenly Father, come into my heart and heal me."

Guiding the car out along the highway, I alternate between bewilderment and deep anger that no one else understands, because Mother now has to face death alone. Her children are around her, but there is no longer any point in talking with her about death. Everyone has put up a barrier and she seems to have done it too. Now in these lonely vigils at her bedside I begin to wonder if that is the way it has to be, and if each of us will go alone. I don't want it to be that way for her. Or me!

Tonight Daniel calls. He tells me about a movie he saw, *Little Big Man*, in which an old Indian chooses a certain day to die.

On that day, he and his adopted son go out and find a very scenic place on the mountain. They spread out his blanket and he lies down upon it, looking out upon the scene he has chosen on his day to die. He closes his eyes and waits to die. There is thunder and then drops of rain. He stands up, wraps his blanket around him, and goes back down the mountain because he will not be rained on when he dies.

That's what Mother is doing. She has come to die and this is the place, but she is not going to be rained on when she dies.

July 19

"I declare your power to the next generation."

Sitting in my old bathrobe, drinking my morning coffee, I
am remembering how easy it is to wrap the prairie around
me like an old bathrobe when I am in need of comfort. And
like my old bathrobe, the prairie is best encountered when
you are alone. It is then that you don't try to explain what
you are feeling. You are alone just to feel, just to be. A good
religion is that way. Silent, powerful, best encountered when
you are alone.

I am convinced that all her life, my Mother's faith was the
first thing she thought about when she awoke at 4 A.M. and
the last thing she considered before she went to sleep at night.
When we were moving some of her things to Helen's this
past spring, I found, written in her still beautiful but now
wavering handwriting on the back of a piece of wrapping
paper, a prayer of David. "Since my youth oh God, you have
taught me. And to this day I declare your marvelous deeds.
Even when I am old and gray, do not forsake me, oh God,
'till I declare your power to the next generation, your might
to all who are to come." She took very seriously David's
advice. Just ask her grandchildren, who received anxious letters about their souls.

After Mother's open-heart surgery in 1986, when she was

recuperating at our Wichita home on Park Place, it was hard to find things for her to do while I was at work. One day I wrote a simple statement on a large piece of paper and asked her to think about each word, then jot down other words that came to mind. She could connect the words and, I said, not knowing if she would do it, "This afternoon when you have time, just make a poem from your collection of thoughts." She had not written poetry for the last few years, but I thought this might bring her comfort.

The phrase I left her was, "The day is beautiful." When I got home at night she had these words branching out from "day": sunshine—fresh air—breathing—resting—no pain—peace— eternal life. These words were connected to "beautiful": gifts—health—power—God—the beginning—foreverness. And then she put them together like this.

> There is sunshine in this day and fresh air around me.
> I am breathing and I am resting.
> There is no pain and there is peace in eternal life.
> Fresh air in this beautiful day brings health
> and the power to do things.
> They are gifts of God who was in the beginning
> and is my foreverness.

Alice Brunner
October 1986

64

I will always remember Mother with the New Testament in her hands, head bowed, poring over each word. It was her forever companion. At night seated with her children around the dining room table, sitting reading to our Father when he became nearly blind, alone in her cottage at Hope by the little reading lamp, and finally, in her room in the hospital. She had read it for almost eighty years.

July 21

Mother moans over and over, "Helen, Helen, oh Helen."
My sister whispers, "Helen is just a household word."

In the midst of mental anguish, Mother calls for Helen, who
worries I am hurt because Mother calls for her instead of
me. So she says, "Helen is just a household word. It's generic."
I tell her I understand. And I do. I understand the deep caring
that has caused her to leave her job to stay with our Mother
as she dies. If I try to thank Helen, she shrugs it off. But the
fact remains, for our Mother, "Helen" has become a generic
term for "love."

Pure, unselfish love is what Helen has given our Mother
these last months of her life. It began several years ago when
Mother became lonely living alone. Helen would be with her
on a regular basis, taking her to Herington and to shop and
eat. Helping her with the washing, taking her to buy groceries, taking the garbage to the city's sanitation plot—those
times became precious to Mother and she looked forward
to them. But it was more than groceries, garbage, or lunch
(all of which could have been done in one afternoon). Helen
spaced those visits so she would show up at Mother's little
house two or three times a week. The highlights of Mother's
last few years were provided by Helen, the caregiver.

Now Helen travels thirty minutes from Durham every day except for Saturday, which she spends with her husband, Tom. So Mother knows no matter how long and lonely the nights, no matter how unsettling the relationship with others around her, Helen will always be there in the morning.

Helen is easygoing, caring, and accepting of people. She makes accidents funny, trivializes the trivial, and has respect for what is important. She is real. If I were to tell her this, she would get a tear in her eye and then make a joke out of it. That's Helen. She can be very exasperating because she doesn't want people to be hurt or unhappy around her, and she'll do almost anything to keep such things from happening. But for many of us, "Helen" is a household word.

One day I saw Helen come in and go over to the shelf to put the clean gown away and then walk over to Mother in her wheelchair, to give her a kiss. Mother's eyes followed her everywhere, and then Helen bent over and put her hands on Mother's arms and said, "Ah Mama, I love you." And Mother's face mirrored the warmth from inside, and she just smiled with love in her eyes. Mother's eyes communicate as well as her voice. Sometimes she says, "Oh, I love you too." Other times she is silent and you read it in her eyes.

Today when I got to the hospital at noon, I could see Mother was feeling a little mischievous. Helen, who had been taking care of her all morning, went out to get some coffee. She was gone about twenty minutes and when she got back she started rubbing Mother's arm while we were talking. Then she turned to Mother and said,

"Ah Mama, I love you. You know that, don't you?"
Mother replied quizzically, "Nooo?"
Helen stopped with a pained expression on her face and asked, "Well, Mama, what more do I have to do?"
And Mother said, "Stand on your head."

July 23

"How are you today, Mother?"
"Not very good. I need to take some medicine now."
"What kind of medicine, Mother?"
"The kind where I choose to get up and where I choose to go to the bathroom."

She is trying to make it humorous, but it is a sad moment for me. She has finally learned to tolerate the catheter, but it was hard. At times, this little hospital room became a comic-relief stage.

Mother: "I have to go to the bathroom."
Helen: "Go ahead and go."
Mother: "Goodbye."
Helen: "I'm going to be right here."

Seconds later.

Mother: "I have to go to the bathroom."
Helen: "Go ahead and go."
Mother: "Goodbye."
Helen: "I'm going to be right here."

Still later.

Mother: "I have to get up."
Helen: "Why?"
Mother: "I have to go to the bathroom."
Helen: "Mother, you have a catheter, a tube into your bladder. If you 'pee' it will go in a little bag."
Mother: "Oh, yes."

Pause.

Helen: "Go ahead and go."
Mother: "Goodbye."

Was she laughing inside? Maybe. And quite possibly. Inability to care for herself has been hard on our fastidious little Mother. One day she had been up and down so much she had worn us all out with false trips to the bathroom. Since the pad on her bed had become soiled, an aide said to her, "Just go ahead and go, we'll clean it up." I saw the look on her face. At that moment, she was beyond humor. She couldn't possibly have done it; it was against everything she was taught.

Later on, when accidents happened, she didn't say a word, just lay there silently while they gently cleaned her. I wanted to scream "NO!" Instead, I cried inside.

July 25

"Are the kids getting enough to eat?"

It is hard to think of things to say as we sit by her bedside. Ordinary things of our lives do not seem important now. She still responds to humor, so I tell Mother about an incident that occurred yesterday.

I found some shirts in a hanging box that hadn't been unpacked since our move from Wichita. One is a pale beige shirt, a color Donavon has been looking for. I gave it a cursory glance and seeing it unwrinkled, I hung it in his closet. Yesterday he found it and put it on. When he came home last night, I gave him a hug. Then I saw something on his shoulder. A spot of paint, almost the color of the shirt but looking suspiciously like a bird had made an unwelcome deposit. "Oh my gosh, Donavon!" I said, knowing he had just come out of a meeting with staff. "Who was sitting to your right?" "Well," he said, with typical Kansas humor, "I really couldn't say. They kept getting up and moving away." When I tell Mother, she smiles.

The afternoon wears on and she is tired. Half asleep, she asks, "Are your kids getting enough to eat?" A little later, she murmurs, "The cats get enough to eat." Farm talk, from thirty years ago, things she had to worry about then.

I sigh, for Mother is starting to disassociate from the familiar present. And she is beginning to distance herself from other relatives and friends. She does not care about anything except having her children around her. I tell Helen, "If we were to stop coming she would die." Helen nods. I could sit beside her, hold her hand, and help her push a button while she dies, but I could never abandon her.

I am disturbed. The disappointments of this day wear on me as I travel I-70 home. Passing a sign, "1 Kansas farmer feeds 92 people and you," I turn again to poetry.

> Are the kids getting enough to eat?
> Will the rain come in time for the wheat?
> I woke up this morning and no longer ask why
> For today is my day to die.

Usually the highway is an avenue through the hills of grass. Today it represents a paved intrusion with attendant bill-boards and clutter. The clutter is most irritating.

> If the president falters again in his task
> If the city hides 'neath its toxic mask
> If someone hurts I won't hear the cry
> For today is my day to die.

Near the Snokomo Road turnoff, I see cottonwoods twirling their leaves in the gentle breeze. They are silent survivors of summer heat and winter ice. I am reminded once again that only the strong survive on the prairie. Mother is no longer strong.

July 26

A Tree Grows on the Prairie

Kasia, my oldest granddaughter, and Tahnoqua, the youngest, are spending the day with me. Eleven-year-old Kasia, sensing that all is not right with my world, spent some quiet time writing "Winds of Love," which ended, "Nothing can stop the wind in my heart from blowing warm into your arms."

Early this morning we went grocery shopping, and as I turned around after getting an item from the shelf, I saw a little girl wrinkle up her nose at Tahnoqua in an obvious act of dislike. Three-year-old Tahne put her arms around me and whispered, "She doesn't know I'm a special Indian princess."

When we got home, I told Tahne (what she already knew) that she was indeed special because she was indigenous—her mother's people were native people. Then I explained that her father's people came from Europe. I drew two family trees for her. A tree for her father, Daniel, and a tree for her mother, Melody. Melody's father was Chippewa and her mother ("Guko" to Tahne) is Mesquakie.

73

"See," I said, "across the crown are small branches for the very earliest ancestors."

"What is that," she asked, pointing to several twigs which ended abruptly.

"They are people whose names we do not know, but they are very important," I said. "If not for them, we would not be here."

On my family tree, the English and Scotch-Irish have the longest branches, then the Swedes, and the very shortest branches are the Germans from Russia who came last to the prairie. Across the breadth of the tree I wrote the names of members of the large families of our early settler ancestors. I explained to my granddaughters how a large family made a farm far more self-sufficient than one that had few children. The Anderson/Falen family had ten children: Aaron, William, Roy, John, Ernest, Rose, Leona, Edward, Viola, and Agnes. I have a cherished family photograph, taken around 1910, of the six brothers standing beside their six Fords. In that same generation, the Robinson/Stacks family had only six children: Charles, Edith, Clara, Harriet, Myrtle, and Cora. It was probably considered a small family.

There were many chores to do to survive on the farm. There were generally more chores than daylight! With the thirteen children of the Brunner/Beisel family—Henry, Amalia, Lydia, Alexander, Eva, Marie, Solomon, Johanna, Daniel, Benjamin, Samuel, David, and Joseph—the labor force was adequate to grow and harvest their food, preserve it, cook it, put it on the table, and clean up afterward. My Grandmother died at a fairly young age—the downside of that story. I never knew her.

So, I showed Tahnoqua how all these families converge at the trunk of the tree. The trunk represents my brother John, sister Helen, and me. The roots twisting and turning through the soil are our children—Lance, Daniel, Robin, Doni Marie, Roger, Robert, Joel, Christina, Alyce, and Joy. Debbie, Richard, and Russell are grafted but firmly attached to the tree.

Roots are a symbolic part of the prairie. Fed and nurtured by fire and decomposition, grass roots bring new life. So on the roots of our family tree are little nubs starting to grow. They are the grandchildren from Joshua down to Joseph Devon. I explain to Tahne that she is one of these nubs.

> "This is our prairie tree," I say, "the old ones across the top branches, the powerful trunk changing with each generation, and the roots forever alive, forever young, like the tall grass."
> Tahnoqua has been bending over my picture of the family tree. "Great-grandmother will soon be up here," she says, pointing to a higher branch.

Joel and Tracy have been visiting. Mother reaches up and touches Joel's face. There is a brightness in her eyes as she whispers, "Joel, as you touch other people, you will bless their lives."

The grandchildren visit on weekends. Today, Mother started talking about the time when Lance, at four years of age, came to visit her and his Grandfather. One morning, hearing Grandmother leave for work, Lanny (as he was called then) leaped out of the bathtub, eluded Grandpa, and ran down to the main street of Hope, dripping wet, his towel held at arm's length in front of him, yelling for his Grandmother! We laugh, remembering. Then she quietly says, "The first one is always a little special, don't you think?"

It was fascinating to me that she could make each grandchild feel special, as if the one who was with her at any given time was her favorite. She bought art supplies for Richard. She knew that Robert liked to play horseshoes. She knew Roger's favorite cartoons and that Robin stored things in a box under her bed. (Once, even a dead bird!) She knew which doll Christina liked best and that Debra wanted to spend time talking. She knew Russell liked to fish. She saved bugs for Daniel's collection. And whenever she could, she participated in their lives. Even last Friday, when Helen told Mother that

Joy, her youngest granddaughter, would be playing in a volleyball game that night, Mother wanted to go. She didn't say anything to Helen, but toward evening when John and Maggie came to the hospital, she raised up in bed and said, "Find my brown pants please, so I can get dressed for the game." John had to convince her that this time she would not be going.

Earlier this morning, Helen told Mother she would be gone for a while but would be only a few blocks away. Helen said, "I'm leaving now, Mother, but I'll be close if I'm needed." Mother replied, with her eyes closed, "Well, you go on, Honey, you go on without me this time."

Mother, who was named for her grandmother, also has a namesake granddaughter. Alice Stacks arrived in Kansas in a covered wagon to become one of the first settlers in Dickinson County. Alice Anderson survived the Great Depression, two world wars, and is dying as the Cold War collapses. Now, Alyce Bishop faces a world filled with threats to the environment and the health of its people. But the models are there. Her grandmothers simply did what they had to do and this Alyce can, too.

July 28

She opens her eyes and begins, "Oh, Ma'am?"
I laugh, "There's no Ma'am here, just Carol."
She closes her eyes, "Yes, lady."

It is becoming more apparent that the staff feels we are unhappy about a lack of pain control and that we blame the
doctor for this. This has created a state of anarchy, with each
shift deciding the kind of medicine, the time given, and even
if Mother is to get it.

I am frustrated that her medical attendants' personal attitudes
about dying are making the decisions about how our Mother
is to spend these last days of her life. The doctor comes and
goes. The people who really act out this high drama of her
life are her children and the nursing staff. We are with her
day in and day out, but the doctor calls the shots (bad pun),
or, more often than not, avoids calling them. One day I told
him Mother was in pain and he said that that is not what he
heard from the staff. What is going on? Why? Why does my
Mother have to die this way? They have made it perfectly
clear they wish she were well enough to be in a nursing home.
Are nursing homes places where people have to go to die?
The thought becomes an obsession with me. Where do we
go to die?

Mother has fallen asleep and I am alone. There is so little to do in this room when Mother is asleep, as she is so often. I doze in my chair, thinking about hospitals all across America trying to keep old dying people out.

In a semisleep, I see the gleaming white of millions of hospitals clustered in front of a gigantic building on which is printed the words Health Care Finance Administration. Inside the building a committee sits, like Madame Defarge at the guillotine, counting the bodies in the hospital morgues. On their right side is a wall labeled "good" and on their left a wall labeled "bad." Once in a while a man rises to write a hospital's name on one of the walls. In horror I realize that "good" and "bad" have nothing to do with the quality of care received in the hospitals. It has only to do with the number of old people who die there.

And now I think of the faces of elderly patients up and down the halls on either side of my Mother. The beautiful, creased, age-lined faces of the people who were the strength of my community when I was a child. There exists, for them, a nationwide "standard mortality formula" that will dictate whether or not they die a dignified death in a hospital setting.

Floating in and out of this dream-like state, I see names on the "bad" wall—mostly little rural hospitals. My people. I wake to the sound of my own voice saying, "Somebody needs to do something about those folks." The sound echoes in this silent room. The idea of even approaching hospital regulators is futile and depressing. Today, for my Mother, dying is walking a road of denial, dependent on and needing medical care, but making do with what she gets.

Now Mother is awake and her agitation is great. I believe it is due to mental stress and the instability of her heart. It is becoming apparent to me she needs some medication for both calming and physical discomfort. Finally, I ring for the nurse and an aide comes in. I tell her I want to talk to an RN about the way Mother is feeling now. One comes immediately. She is from Hope and has cared for both our Father and Mother. She knows the family history. Now she stays and talks about the effect of drugs. I say to her, "All her life Mother has been unable to sleep and this is compounding her current distress. I am not comfortable with the doctor telling us she is in no pain. If he believes that, is she getting the right medicine?" This nurse, with much compassion in her face, explains very kindly and carefully their procedures, but the explanations do not satisfy.

Aunt Helen, Mother's sister, calls from Illinois. Mother's voice is strong and she is able to make herself heard to Aunt Helen. Later on, Helen Rose comes and sits silently by Mother's side. I hear Helen whisper and I turn to see that Mother is rubbing

Helen's arm like she used to when we were little. Helen looks up with shining eyes.

I leave the hospital for the journey home. I am nervous and angry and I want to fix this dying. I want to make it right. Just one mile north of the hospital, I am in the midst of prairie and it demands my attention.

The sun is going down and as it sinks toward the horizon, it becomes larger and larger until it is an enormous flattened orb. All around me is gold and crimson as the sun slides down the sky. It is going fast. A kaleidoscope of colors shines before me with the hills bathed in lavender. On one side is dark and shadow, on the other is light and distinct lines.

The moon will come up tonight and when it is just on the horizon the reverse will occur. A large, almost unreal prairie moon, as if a child took a paintbrush and made an exaggeration on the canvas of our sky, will move up the sky until it becomes its rightful size once more.

Will the distortion of my Mother's dying even out some day? Maybe, but for now, back in her little room, she is making do with what she gets.

July 29

"Her laughter lies for her now and pats our backs."
Doni Marie

Today, I see Mother is in pain so I call the nurse and tell her.

She asks "Are you having pain, Alice?"
Mother replies, with a sigh, "Oh, no."
I immediately ask, "Can you tell us where it
hurts, Mother?"
"Yes, here," and she points across her chest.

Mother tries so hard to please everyone, and she says what she thinks she should say or what she thinks they want her to say. Add that to the stoicism she inherited from her father and her seventy-nine years of practice at hiding her discomfort. This combination makes it difficult for her to request what she really needs from her medical providers. I try to explain our mother to the nurses. But there is no place for such a notation on the chart.

John told me last night that when he and Maggie were there, an LPN came in with medications. Knowing Mother likes this particular nurse, John asked, "Mother, isn't this the good nurse?" And Mother, looking at the woman mixing all the medicines together in a cup of Metamucil and Jell-O, replied, "Yes, she's a good nurse, but she doesn't make good food."

In the evening, back in Topeka, I get a phone call from Doni Marie, a performance artist, in Berlin, Germany. She asks me to tell Grandma that more than anything, she hopes she is not afraid. She says she loves her very much and always has a picture of her and Grandpa with her. I will faithfully repeat all this to Mother. In looks and actions, they are much alike. Doni went to her with her growing-up problems and Grandma always listened. Through the years Doni found Grandma didn't criticize but would make plain what she thought about the situation and then accept Doni's different interpretation. I, on the other hand, often tried to protect Mother from knowing about worrisome situations. Once Doni said to me, "Mother, quit tiptoeing around Grandma. She may be little in size, but she is strong in spirit."

Sometimes I think my Mother vicariously lived some of her own dreams through Doni. When Doni Marie graduated from high school in the 1970s, she sneaked skates into the auditorium and then, to the delight of her classmates, she roller-skated across stage to receive her diploma! Shaking hands with the school board president, she used his hand to propel herself across the stage into the arms of a laughing (thank goodness!) principal. We did not know whether to sneak out or applaud. A member of the family leaned over to us and said, "If she were my daughter, she would skate home tonight." But Grandmother Alice sat quietly, unabashed pride all over her face. I will never forget Mother's reaction.

Doni Marie, in her own pain at being far away while Grandma is dying, writes to me. She is aware that Mother's humor has sustained us through this very long summer.

Now, in tiny letters on a foreign postcard, carried by a stamp bearing an unfamiliar face across the forests and ocean and cities between us, come the haunting words of my daughter.

> Mother, dear Mother, you ask of me a letter.
> The least a daughter can do for a Mother
> An ocean, a continent, a world away.
> There in my Mother's land lies her Mother
> In some undignified chamber rotting slowly
> But still laughing for her daughter's sake.
> Her laughter lies for her now and pats our backs . . .
>   Doni Marie
>   Berlin 1991

Undated in July

"He [the doctor] knows how I hurt in my heart."

The limit to her endurance has finally come. Mother can no longer be brave. She has been restless all morning, so I don't go to lunch until the middle of the afternoon. When I return, Mother says to me, "It hurts in here, oh it hurts. Jesus is coming." I tell her, "If it hurts Mother, let's call the nurse for some medicine." It is 4:45 P.M. Mother looks at me and says, "I told the nurse I needed something strong and she said I had to wait until seven." Three hours? No! This will not do.

An aide is standing beside the bed. Sensing my anger, she says, "Just pick up that phone. Just pick up that phone and call the doctor. You have to call the doctor." She leaves and I watch her go, grateful for the support. I call the clinic and talk to the doctor over his walk phone. He says Mother's heart is in bad condition and it won't be long now. I tell him "That's not why I'm calling. I want her to have something stronger." He tells me he will talk to the nurse. About five minutes later, I am summoned to the phone in the nurses' station. The doctor says he is getting conflicting messages. The nurse tells him Mother isn't in pain, she is only moaning. I tell him, with rigid jaw, "I've sat by her since eleven this morning and they've just been in and out." He reminds me I am not a professional. I ignore this. We both know I am not a medical person. I try again, telling him that "her pain is different now and I want you to see her, now." He says "Okay, I'll come."

I go back into Mother's room and the first words I hear are "It hurts." She has been stoic and uncomplaining all this time. It's inconceivable no one will hear her now. The respiration therapist comes in to do a treatment. I worry Mother will be better when the doctor comes but she isn't. He comes in with a nurse and standing across the bed from me, starts telling me about Medicare regulations! He says it will be murder to give Mother heavy dosages of pain medication. I look at him and wonder if he knows that this hospital's reports have become more important than my Mother. Perhaps it really is not his fault. In the medical profession, quality means life. And it is not his fault that such an attitude creates blatant discrimination against old people. On the contrary, he cares very much for these folks.

But now I feel it's time to do battle. The doctor may have to play games with the regulators, but I don't have to and I am here to see that my Mother does not suffer because some faraway, foolish officials think they can set a standard for death. He affirms he cannot give Mother any more pain medicine until seven. He goes on to say her heart is getting weaker and weaker and will eventually go.

Literally in tears and without censoring my conversation, I ask,

"And when her heart goes, are we going to withhold pain medication because it isn't seven o'clock or whatever the time will be then?"

For the first time, he turns and looks at Mother. Panicky, I ask her to tell him how she feels. In a weak voice she says,

"He knows, he knows how I hurt in my heart."
I can tell it has an impact on him. He asks me,
"Do you want a drip of morphine?"
I ask, "Is that best for her?"
He says, "It will be constant and not up and down."

I agree to it and he leaves. I feel an enormous sense of relief.

Later that evening

"She's just going to bottom out."

All hell has broken loose. You think the doctor and the patient and her children can make this decision? There is the nursing staff yet to contend with. I go down the hall to use the pay phone and come back to see John, who has just entered the hospital, accosted by a nurse who is saying, "She's just going to bottom out—just bottom out. I don't want to be responsible for her death."

Back in Mother's room, several nurses come in and look at her. One says, "I won't be able to find a vein." I don't stay to watch and the nurse was right, they can't find a vein. So they put the morphine in the existent IV and her arm begins to swell. The IV has to be taken out and the nurse who had not wanted her on morphine throws down her gloves and says, "Let the doctor do it. He wants it, let him do it."

At 7:30 P.M. the doctor comes in and puts the needle in her arm with a board to hold it stationary. At 9:20 I stop by the nurses' station to talk to a nurse writing her report. She says to me, "See, you can't tell any difference, she's still agitated." I remind her that I can tell a difference—a big one: Mother isn't in pain. I am certain she did not include what I said in her report.

I now have no credibility with the nursing staff. Helen tells me they truly want what is right for her. I know that. They probably thought I just wanted her kept quiet. I did want her to be able to sleep, but most of all I didn't want her to suffer. I had promised Aunt Helen I would see Mother didn't suffer. And most important, I did something no one else did: I believed Mother when she finally told us she was hurting.

I leave the hospital at 9:45 with the feeling that the nurses are trying to protect my Mother from me! It makes me glad and mad at the same time. I ask John and Maggie to stay with Mother until I am gone, for it has become increasingly difficult to leave her when no one is there. They agree. I kiss the top of her head and tell her our childhood parting, "See you in the morning, Mother." She nods.

When I leave the hospital for the drive home through the black hills and the brilliant stars, things are again in proper perspective. I am one small part of this universe and I did what I was called upon to do. Now I can let it go.

In the night with the rush of wind past my car and the hills fading one into another, I release the weight of my decision and begin to pray, "It is in your hands. Let her go quietly and quickly if it is her time to die. And if it is not her time, then let it be. I was just doing the best I knew how when no one else was doing a thing."

I talk to John and Maggie the next day. They say she slept last night and is peaceful and at rest. Later on, Helen calls. She says Mother is not agitated and I did the right thing. I am vindicated. Mother did not "bottom out."

July 31

"Eat, Alice, so you can get well and go home!"

I have just come down the long hills through the prairie
morning brightness. I find my Mother sitting up in a chair.
The nurse is so proud she is sitting up. "Look," she says to
me. "Isn't it wonderful?" It's obvious she has been telling
Mother again that she has to eat to get well. I look at the
brightness in Mother's eyes and see this false hope is getting
through. They have worked a small miracle again.

When the nurse leaves, Mother asks, "Am I better?"
She knows I won't lie to her. "What do you mean?" I ask.
"Is my body getting better?"
"No, Mother." All I can offer is love. Let it be enough.

I am amazed. These people who deal so positively with living
could deal positively with dying. Why don't they? I know it is
hard to have a patient die, especially one who is well known
to the staff. But what medical school teaches a denial of death?   91
This denial, and its attendant deceit, has made Mother's
dying a nightmare.

The nurses have told me Mother's doctor is a perfectionist
who has difficulty seeing his patients die. I remember for the
last five years of Mother's life, if she got hurt at home (one
time she broke her arm) and we had to take her for medical

help to his office, he seemed to think the accident was our fault for letting her live alone. We were glad then he was so protective of her. We were all secure in knowing she had such good medical care. So what happened? He can't fix it this time.

When Mother asks "Am I getting well?" why don't these medical people come in, sit down by her side, take her hand, and explain that her body is wearing out, that they will make her comfortable and be with her as she dies? The inability of others to be supportive of her dying has created problems for me. I have begun to wonder if I have done the wrong thing these last few weeks. Would she have gotten well if we had taken her to a cardiologist in Wichita? What if she could have gotten better with different medical attention a month ago? And what if I've been saying to her, Mother you are dying, when in fact, she isn't? Last week, I was almost devastated by this thought. I asked Donavon, as I always do when I am not sure about reality, "Would the doctor have told us she was dying if she wasn't?" He assured me he would not have done such a thing.

This morning I look at her and she is strong, her color is good. Again she looks directly into my eyes and says, "I want to ask the doctor if there has been a change in my body. Do I need to see a specialist?"

"Okay, we will ask the doctor." I go out to the nurses' desk to see if Mother's doctor has already made his rounds. He has, so I get his number and ask his office to have him call me when he can.

A nurse comes in. I tell her Mother wants to know if she is getting better. The nurse says, "Her kidneys are better." This is one of the nurses who has been saying to this dying patient, "You have to eat so you will get better." I look at her and think the events of this day are a result of her little deception.

Soon the doctor arrives. I tell him what Mother is wanting to know. He says, "No, there is no change." When pressed further, he says she will have to go to Wichita if she wants to see a heart doctor. I ask Mother if she understands and I repeat part of it, for he was talking softly. Then he leaves.

It is silent in the room for a long time. Finally Mother dejectedly says,

<blockquote>
"Lets get rid of the doctor."
"Why, Mother?"
"We don't need him anymore."
</blockquote>

She looks tired and depressed. I call a nurse and she is put back into bed. After a while she turns to me and says,

"I want to go home."
"To your house in Hope?"
"No."
"To Helen's house?"
"No."
"To John's house?"
"No."

We are quiet for a while. Then I ask her,

"Do you mean your heavenly Father's home?"
She replies, "Yes, it is time to go."

I want to run away and cry. But I find the strength to say,

"In His own time, Mother, in His own time."

She nods. She understands, of course.

I will always remember this as the day they stole from my Mother. It could have been a celebration of a beautiful life now almost over. They could have said, "Isn't it wonderful you have this beautiful day, Alice?" Instead they said she was getting better. And when she realized what they had done, the reality of her impending death was overpowering.

AUGUST

August in Kansas is about waiting

Waiting for the growing season to end
Waiting for the last field's yield
Waiting for the coming of winter
Waiting for the earth to sleep.

So the green turns brown
And the stalks bend down.
The cattle forage low
And the heat hangs around.

The rain has stopped
And the windmills pump
Everyone waits
While time   moves   slow.

August in Kansas is about waiting.

ON THE
PRE-AGRARIAN
PRAIRIE

Third Scene

On a certain evening, after the sun goes home over the horizon and darkness moves over the land, a lone coyote mounts the tallest hill, throws back its head, and sends a mournful cry across the tall grass. As if in answer, clouds appear on the horizon. They flow across the sky, building higher and higher into massive thunderheads. Below, a slight ripple moves the dying grass. Electricity charges the air, bolts flash down the sky dome. Energy is unleashed in streaks of brilliance. Prairie creatures, bodies tingling, are driven out of holes and from under cliffs to see, feel, and cower back.

Lightning zaps the ground with increased vigor. Across the hills comes a rolling ball of fire. Wind pushes the fire up one hill and down the next. The bison and the antelope, the wolf and the coyote, the hawk and the eagle, the prairie dog and the jackrabbit flee. Some escape, some do not. Blackened hills wait as the fire rushes on.

FROM THE DIARY
IN AUGUST

August 1

> I think she cannot speak and so I say it for her,
> "I love you and you love me."
> "Oh," she says clearly, "I cannot tell you how much."

Today would have been Mother and Daddy's fifty-seventh
wedding anniversary. On their last anniversary together in
1979, Daddy lay dying. We lived in Wichita then, and three
of our four children were still at home when they weren't
in college.

It had started in May. Coming home from a shopping trip, we
were met at the door by Lance. "Grandpa had a stroke" . . .
stroke . . . stroke . . . The word reverberated through my head.
Fear. Adrenalin. Action. I called the hospital and asked to
speak to Mother. She told me it had happened in the middle
of the morning while she was at work.

We'd been warned he could have a stroke at any time since
he'd had one three years earlier, and in the last few weeks he
had begun to beg Mother not to go to work. Premonition,
perhaps.

He was in the garden, this farmer who loved the earth and its creatures, who fifteen years before had gone blind and had to move from the farm to the little town of Hope, who salvaged what he could of his career with a plot of garden behind the house. This year he had planted row after wriggly row of beans. And he did it the only way he could, down on his knees with his one partially sighted eye squinting down the row. Planting is what he had done every year for three-fourths of a century.

His nemesis was the sun. He had fought the sun and the drought and carried bucket after bucket of water pumped from the windmill or pulled from the stock tank. His battle with the sun had spanned decades of fighting its merciless rays, but on this day, the sun triumphed. Daddy fell in the garden and lay with its heat beating down on him.

Sometime later, he stirred and crawling to the fence, pushed himself up from the hard earth. He thought someone had hurt him—had robbed him. He went to the house, searching. Wandering from room to room calling "Alice! Alice!" he found no one. Something was wrong and he did not know what it was. And in the bathroom, he fell again.

At noon Mother went home. Hearing things falling, she ran to the bathroom door, but it was locked. She pleaded with him to unlock the door, but he would not. He was angry, hitting with his fist, pacing like a caged animal in that small

space. In the midst of his confusion, some small remembrance occurred and he reached for and unlocked the door.
He stumbled out past his wife, calling again in terror, "Alice!
Alice!" From room to room in the cottage he walked, with
Mother right behind him saying, "Dan, I'm here." But even
when she stood in front of him, in danger from his swinging
arms, he could not see her.

Frightened, she called a neighbor, who called another and
another, and when it was evident no one knew what else to
do, they called the town marshal. The marshal and three
strong men put their friend into a straitjacket and took him
to the hospital, a place he'd only been in once before in his
life. They tied this three-hundred-pound man to the bed with
wrist and ankle restraints. The doctor came and said to Alice
and the other frightened relatives who had gathered there,
"He does not know anything. He does not know what we are
doing or saying." And my Father saw the congregated family
and felt the leather straps that bound him.

After three days it became apparent he was not going to die
immediately. He fought the restraints and he fought the attendants. Once he hit Mother. His language was garbled and
sometimes the German words of his childhood were inter-
spersed with the English of his adulthood. From time to time
I could almost make sense of some of the sentences, but it
seemed the nouns were missing. He would plead "Help me!
Help me!" and beg with his eyes to have his children cut the

bonds from him. Once he woke and thought he was back on the farm. He begged John to help him get over the fence (bed rail).

All that hot summer, I drove the 180-mile round trip with a triumphant sun overhead. "He can't live much longer," they said. Then they said "He'll live, but he won't ever go home."

One day it was clear to Mother he was calling for me. I drove to the hospital and when everyone left the room, I took his hand and said, "Daddy, they tell me you've been asking for me." He raised himself up, braced against those restraints and began to talk. The veins swelled out on his neck, his eyes became urgent, insistent, his body tense. I listened and none of the words made sense. My head pounded and began to ache. What was it my Father, in his dying, needed to say? In the middle of this agony, a thought screamed out at me: "What am I going to tell him in return?"

Then suddenly he stopped talking and, still braced against the restraints, waited for my answer. I said, "It's all right Daddy. It's all right." And the light went out of his eyes, and he fell back on his pillow and turned his head away from me. In a moment when he needed me as he had never needed me before, I failed my Father. I knew I had done so, and I know it to be one of the greatest mistakes of my life. I should have told him I couldn't understand a thing he was saying. He could understand us and he could think clearly, but when he tried to speak it was all mixed up. I should have. But there was no one to help us understand.

For years, I thought I let our Father die without telling him we could not understand him. Then one day Daniel told me that he was sitting beside Grandpa and heard the mixed-up German/English words. He asked Grandpa if he wanted to go to the bathroom, received an affirmative, and helped him to the bathroom and then back to bed. As he sat there holding his hand, he said to him, "Grandpa, I know you can hear me." Grandpa's eyes snapped alert, and he looked directly at Daniel. Then Daniel said, "I know you're trying to talk to us, but what you are saying is jumbled up and we don't understand." Grandpa squeezed Daniel's hand so hard he thought it would break. He did know, after all.

Finally, toward the end of our Father's last days, I went home to Wichita, my sister went to West Virginia, my brother went to work in Abilene, and they put Daddy in a nursing home. By then his speech was better. "I want to go home," he would beg Mother and John. Daniel, his namesake, offered to give up the next semester of college to stay with him, but Mother made the decision not to keep him at home. She was afraid he might get on the railroad tracks and get hit by a train or burn the house down or do something to embarrass the neighbors.

I only saw my Father three times in the nursing home. There are no words to describe how it felt to see him with that dull drug glaze on his face, begging, "Let's go home, okay?" Mother went every day to sit beside him. Then one day, he tore the curtains from the windows and the sheets off his bed. When Mother got there, they told her they couldn't keep him any longer. She went into his room and sat by his side and rubbed his head until he went to sleep. When he woke, he reached up, took her hand and said, "Pray for me, Alice."

Before we could make alternative arrangements for his care, the doctor discovered Daddy had prostate trouble so he was taken back to the hospital for an operation. He recognized the nurses and his surroundings and was glad to be back among friends.

Mother went home the night he was moved and picked the last of the summer beans. She canned them the next day before going to the hospital. The nursing home had been a horrible mistake.

Life kept going on for us. I had to leave in the middle of a rehearsal dinner for Lance and M'Liz's wedding, because Daddy had gotten worse. And then they were married. I said "Daddy, Lance is married." It fell on deaf ears. His breathing came and went, his strong heart battled, and we admired our frail giant.

Finally, Helen came back. He had been waiting on her, I believe. After spending sixteen hours at the hospital, I was relieved to see her come, and I went home to Wichita on the bus. I desperately needed to rest. I'll never forget how dirty the world looked. The hills I loved were grimy, the roads dusty, the city gritty on the lonesome ride home.

I lay down to rest for a while, intending to go back in the evening. I slept and no one woke me. But at midnight I heard the telephone and made my way down the hall to the library. The phone was not on the desk. Earlier, Joel had taken it into the closet, to sit on the floor while he talked to a teenage friend in private, and left it there. The phone continued its raucous ringing, while in the dark, I crawled toward it on the floor, all the while knowing what the message would be. "He is gone."

I kept a jar of beans from his last crop for many years. It sat on the back of the canned goods shelf, and each time I cleaned, I held it, remembered, and put it back. Ten years later, on the day we moved from Wichita, I left it behind.

I rouse myself from these painful memories. I look at Mother lying there so still, so quiet. What is she remembering? The good, the bad, the fun, the difficult times?

August 3

Tall-grass Women

Today I visit with Mother a while and then tell her that I am going to Hope to attend the funeral of her longtime friend, the mother of my longtime friend. Our families have associated for a century. Mother doesn't seem to want to talk or to think about it. She is preoccupied—or maybe remembering.

Alice May and Ruby May were both born in 1912. They went through school together, attended the same church together, enjoyed youth together, and both eventually married. When they had baby daughters, both born in 1938, they named them Carol Marie and Maisie Marie. Maisie and I went to the same school and the same church as our mothers. But unlike our mothers, when we graduated from high school in the late 1950s we left the community. Our mothers always lived in or around Hope; both were widowed for some time; and both suffered heart problems in their old age. Now my Mother is dying at seventy-nine years of age, and Ruby is being buried on her eightieth birthday.

As I drive the roller coaster road to Hope, I realize that I am not going to the funeral to say goodbye to my Mother's friend or my friend's mother (as I have alternately thought of her all these years). I am going to say goodbye to my friend, Ruby. I think of all the tragedy in her life: two grandchildren burned to death, another granddaughter murdered. And I think about how unfair life is. But Ruby, always smiling, always concerned about others, stood in the midst of hardship like prairie tall grass. She bent with the wind and was sometimes laid horizontal to the earth, but she always stood again.

At the funeral, which is widely attended by Hope folks, I look at Maisie and think what she has meant to my life. For thirty-five years we have corresponded only occasionally. We have aged apart, and yet we still think alike. I will always remember the day Maisie brought her teenage daughter home for burial, how we stood in the wind at the cemetery and listened to Maisie read from scripture. She affirmed that she did not have to avenge her daughter's death and claimed the promise that vengeance belonged to God. It was obvious that in spite of her unbelievable grief, Maisie was not going to let herself be consumed with hatred. She comforted us and we admired her for it.

Now I am thinking of the song we sang when we graduated in 1956, "Moments to Remember" by Stillman and Allen. "Though summer turn to winter and the present disappears, the laughter we were glad to share will echo through the years. . . . we will have these moments to remember." And now Maisie's mother is dead and mine is dying, and there is no generation between us and death. Ah Maisie, just when did summer turn to winter?

After the funeral, Maisie and I have only a brief chance to talk. She reminds me that in losing both her daughter and her mother she has lost both her future and her past. So for her there is now only the present. Returning to the hospital, I reflect on what Maisie said. Once I get beyond the loneliness of her words, I realize she is talking about survival. She is a tall-grass woman, and she is going to be okay because right now, there is no other way to be.

August 6

> Mother says quietly, "Someday I'm going to bake bread—
> but not today."

It is a bright hot morning and I am stopped on Highway 77
at a construction site. With my windows rolled down, I sit in
sultry heat, waiting on the flag carrier. This road takes me
south across the breadth of the hills through farm country
and I wait near a prairie-cum-pasture. It has not been burned
in so long that cedar trees have not only invaded but gotten a
good growth. I am irritated at the unknown owner, who is
not a good caretaker of the prairie.

Waiting impatiently in my car, with an oil tanker, several
farm trucks, and a few cars behind me, I think of how this
area would have looked a century and a half ago. I remember
hearing stories about the first pioneers who came to Kansas.
Starting across at the jumping-off place in the beautiful wood-
ed areas of eastern Kansas, often in wagons pulled by slow
oxen, they were ill prepared for what they would encounter.
There was, I believe, plenty of advice on taking trails where
there was water. So, they would heed it and follow an old
trail, or not heed it and just set out in a westerly direction.
But once they left "civilization" behind, reality set in—reality
in the form of an endless grassland stretching before them.

Eventually, some of them became phobic. There was nothing to fix their eyes upon, to let them know that by the next day they would reach a certain mountain or by the evening get to the river, or see the seashore. There was nothing there but grass and hills, and when you topped those hills, there was more of the same. There was only one thing to do. Continue. On and on over the endless prairie. Some succeeded and some failed, depending on the "stuff" of which they were made. Some became so frightened of the aloneness they turned around and went back. They didn't know how to look at the prairie. They had not learned, as Tahne counseled, to "just open their eyes."

There are still people like that today, just as ignorant and just as phobic as they cross the prairie on four-lane I-70. They go for hundred of miles and miss it all.

When I get to the hospital, I find Mother under the influence of a drug. She begins to talk and I bend down. "Let's say we forgive each other and not ask why." I am surprised and I say, "Well, I think that's a good idea." She does not pursue it and goes to sleep. I walk out into the hall and a housekeeper stops and tells me, "Your Mother's life is a testimony to me." As we part, she says quietly, "I pray for her."

When I go back in the room, Mother is awake. I say to her, "I love you Mother." She returns, "I love you, too." Then with a big grin, "I love you three." In the evening we say goodbye and I start out to the car. Realizing I have forgotten the fruit Helen left in a sack for me, I slip back into her room and hear her praying, "Take care of Carol."

August 7

> "Mother," I ask her, " did you enjoy those years on the
> farm?"
> "It was a lot of work," she says. Then with a faraway
> look in her eyes, "I enjoyed the sunsets."

Traveling west out of Topeka on my way to the hospital, I
see an imposing house on the south side of I-70 at the very
top of the hill. What a view there must be up there. And
what a contrast to the old farmhouses of my youth, which
were built down in the draws or on the sides of hills or
cocooned in a shelter belt.

On the way through Junction City to Herington, I think about
how people have lived on the prairie. First the round grass
huts of the Caddoans, who were here long before the Europeans came. Their descendants, the Wia-chi-toh, lived in winter lodges of grass and in summer tepees of bison hides.
There is a certain place near Matfield Green on the Kansas
Turnpike that lies sheltered between the hills. A slender
stream makes its way down the valley. It has the look and feel
of a place where the native people might have stayed during
winter. I have no way of knowing, and perhaps it is just a fan-
tasy, but each time I pass that place, I am aware of something
I cannot name.

The art of native people was functional. It was woven into

their clothing, beaded on their moccasins, painted onto the sides of the tepees, imprinted on their utensils. To my knowledge, nobody said they should leave art to the "artists" as we do today.

The first homes of the Europeans were dugouts with wood fronts and bison-skin doors built into the side of a hill and sod houses built of squares of prairie sod cut and carefully fitted on top of each other, with cottonwood poles laid across the top, holding up more sod squares for the roof. They were very functional dwellings for the prairie.

Mother once told me how my greatgrandparents Robinson lived when they first came to the prairie. Greatgrandmother Alice was always embarrassed about having lived in a loft above their stock. But the stock provided extra heat that first winter when they almost didn't survive.

A generation later, my grandparents Anderson lived in two rooms over two rooms with shutters on the windows to keep out the hail. Close by the back door was a cellar where food was stored that provided safety during tornadoes. A stack of wood in the yard was kept almost as tall as the house. As the family prospered, they built onto their home.

In another generation, my parents lived in a typical prairie farmhouse, the kind that is vanishing today but which sprang up all across Kansas at the turn of the century, partly because they were sold through the Sears catalog. They were two rooms over two rooms with a large room to the side and a porch on either side of it. Our home had a cistern on the back porch and a cellar door connected to the front porch. A well-worn path led to the toilet. A well was located closer to the barn than the house.

After the turn of the century, the "prairie square" came into being. Patterned after the work of architects Green and Green, it was basically four huge rooms over four rooms, with a full basement and, in city homes a third-floor ballroom. The country farmhouses patterned after this style were usually large but not so elaborate. The houses were built for the prairie—to take advantage of the prevailing breezes. They had several balconies on which to sleep in hot weather and a front porch where family members sat and visited. Donavon and I raised our family in such a home on Park Place in Wichita.

In the 1920s, the airplane bungalow, designed for the medium-income family, was built in the cities of Kansas. Most of the living area was downstairs. The two bedrooms, located at the back of the top floor to catch prevailing winds, made it shaped like an airplane.

Now I sit in this modern hospital, watching my Mother sleep, thinking that there has not been a prairie house, with the exception of some Frank Lloyd Wright homes, since the 1920s. Now, we build like our coastal cousins. We take off the porches and go inside to use switches for climate, television for news, and alarms for security. We build fences to become separate from each other and, if we can, we build on top of windswept, treeless hills with windows that do not open. They are great energy wasters, built for the vista alone.

But the old farm folks on those long-ago family farms left their homes in the protection of the draw and climbed a hill for a view. My Mother walked west past the apricot grove and north of the barn to the pasture to watch the sunset. Things did not come easy to prairie dwellers, and they never expected them to. And when they had walked those extra yards and climbed those extra hills, they had earned their view.

Early August

Hold the Halcion

The confusion has continued. John sees it the most, because
he is there in the evening when she is tired from the day. Last
night when he got to the hospital, Mother whispered, "John,
John, things haven't been going too well." Then, seeing a
nurse enter, she whispered conspiratorially, "Shh, I'll tell
you later."

Today, she wakes startled, and seeing the table by the door,
says, "Push that out. Just push that out in the hall." Since it is
the table that holds her food, I decide it is needed here and
try to change her focus, but she keeps coming back to it.
Finally I say,

> "We can't push it out in the hall."
> "Why?"
> "Because they won't like it."
> She is silent a moment considering, then
> matter-of-factly says,
> "Well, we won't worry about that. Just push it out
> and close the door."
> So I do.

Last night John said she thought a cat was in the hospital, and it kept going by the door. John said she prayed about it, so he knew it was bothering her. Mother never wanted cats in the house. Last night, when John got ready to leave, she said, "Take the cat with you." "Okay Mother," he said, "I'll pick it up in the hall."

They have been giving her Halcion to help her sleep. All her life she has been a light sleeper at night and unable to sleep at all during the day. She also has a sensitivity to drugs. Now I worry about the Halcion, which was recently banned in Great Britain.

Sitting beside Mother, I think Halcion won't be banned here until the pharmaceutical company has made as much as they possibly can from it. That's the way we do things. My thoughts go back to a food supplement I took this morning. The Food and Drug Administration wants to control that, also. Not necessarily for my good or for the small entrepreneur's gain. A society is sick when its medical services and drugs are entrapped by money. Now I feel silent anger again. At least today my anger has a new name, Halcion.

There is a very concerned nurse on tonight's shift, who says, "The Halcion is not doing her any good and could be creating problems for her. I've decided to hold the Halcion." I laughingly say, "That would be a good title for a book." My laughter hides my concern, for I fear Mother is hooked on the drug and faces more anxiety and depression when she goes off of it. How can we know which symptoms are caused by the heart and which are caused by the drug? The nurse leaves. Mother is in prayer, "Heavenly Father, I forgive you for making things miserable for me." Later, she begins a chant.

Mother: (moaning) "Helen, Helen, Helen."
Helen: (gently) "Mother . . ."
Mother: "What? WHA-TA?" (with a little push of air to emphasize the final T)
Helen: "Did you want me, Mother?"
Mother: "I guess so."

Seconds later.

Mother: "Helen, Helen, Helen."
Helen: "Here I am, Mother."
Mother: (in surprise) "WHA-TA?"
Helen: "Did you want me, Mother?"
Mother: (confused) "I guess so."

I believe her confusion between knowing she is going to die and wanting to stay alive is exaggerated by the people around her. Her prayers showed us the extent of her confusion: "Heavenly Father, guide me, don't let me go away," then incredibly, "I don't trust you, I don't trust you."

For the last few moments, in her dream state, she has been making a pie. Now, opening her eyes, she asks something I never heard before in this long summer: "Carol, stay with me a little while." I stay longer tonight. Later on, in her prayers, I hear " . . . that I might go to sleep and be yours now. Amen." I watch her closely and hear her pray, "Guide me, take care of me, like you would a child." It is disconcerting. I tell her I am going out to get a can of pop and will be right back. Half awake, she says, "Maybe it will help you sleep. Lots of times, sleeping helps a person." She badly wants to sleep.

Her supper is brought in and I dread seeing it come. When Helen is here, she feeds her, but often one of the aides does the feeding. One day last week, I arrived after she was fed and she started complaining about her lip. I found food stuffed up around her gums and I shuddered with repulsion. Someone was pushing the spoon in again and again, sticking it way into the back of her mouth. Globs of Metamucil had hardened against the roof of her mouth. I knew it was painful. When I told Helen about it, she said quietly, "That is not good nursing." It was the first time I heard her say anything negative about the nursing care.

Today, I got into an argument about the amount of food she is to be given. The nurse's aide tried to explain to me: "If we don't feed her, then we are starving her to death." I explain what I learned after my husband had his heart attack: if a person is overfed, the blood flow to the stomach to aid digestion will take circulation from the heart. I don't like to see her get so much. She is small and completely inactive, and she is used to eating small amounts. What I say makes little difference. They are going to do what they want because they equate eating with living, and they want her to live. They do not believe that dying is a part of living.

On the way home, I think how I like things orderly and well timed. A good life is mostly a matter of timing. In the passages of my life, in the traditions of the family, I like things to be orderly and not awkward. Mother's dying is becoming awkward.

August 10

I bend down to give Mother a hug and am reminded
again of the curious way these sheets smell. I think of her
sheets with the smell of summer upon them. A clean,
windswept smell. "Do you remember?" I ask her. "Uum,"
she murmurs and goes back to sleep.

I am six. There is wind through my hair and sun on my face.
I reach up, grab hold of the wire, and lift my tanned feet from
the hard, packed earth. Swinging back and forth, a sheet slaps
me on one side, sloppy wet towels on the other. Back and
forth. Back and forth. Then comes her call, "Don't hang on
the line, please."

How did she know? I always waited until the first line was
full of sheets before I began my swing on the second line. I
thought I was well hidden, because the second line was
reserved for the things we did not want anyone else to see.
And oh, the lines made tempting swings. No little piece of
rope for us—we had a big stubborn wire. It took a strong
person to stretch it taut when it became loose from wind
and children. Sometimes it had to be propped in the middle
with a tall pole, which itself would sway back and forth as
the wind whipped the sheets. I can still see those sheets fly
up and over in a tangle around the wire.

121

In winter, we placed boards under the line and wore boots to hang clothes. We needed a lot of line when all of the clothes had to be out at the same time, for they would take hours to dry. On many a cloudy day, after the clothes froze on the line, we brought them in and dried them around the stove. I remember wrestling Daddy's stiff-frozen overalls from the line to the house. Rarely did we wait for the weather to change before we washed. Important things like tea towels and underclothes had to be kept washed no matter what.

It was not unusual for a sudden Kansas rain to soak down a whole line of dried clothes. Often we came home from town with storm clouds looming over us and pulled into a neighbor's drive to take her wash down from the line and put it on her back porch. Then we rushed home to save our own.

On nice sunny summer days, Mother would fold clothes at the line. She would snap them to make sure no wasps or bees were inside the folds, and then, arms held away from her body, fold them the way she put them on the beds, precisely even and flat. That night, we would slide between sheets into that heavenly smell and the softness imparted by the wind and sun.

We saved the best sheets and towels "in case company comes" —somebody special like Aunt Helen or Uncle Howard or the minister. And everything was recycled when it was worn out. It was Daddy's undershorts (which made good washcloths) that got Mother into trouble one day. Reverend Jordan had come to talk to her when she was washing dishes and that is how, while emphasizing a point, her hands came up out of the soapy water and in them were Daddy's shorts! Rising to the occasion, Mother looked from shorts to minister and said, "It's been a long time since they were worn."

I glance at her now. She has forgotten I am here. Shadows lengthen outside our window and I am chilled. My reverie is finished. I will never go home again to sleep in a bed where the sheets smell like sun and wind.

In the winter, on a Sunday night, Mother would call
Grandpa Anderson. "Hello Poppa, what does the weather look like for wash day tomorrow?"
"Cold but sunny" is what she wanted to hear.

Kansans often remark, "You don't like our weather? Just wait
a minute." We do experience it all and sometimes in the same
day. We are people, after all, who have at times stood in the
sun and watched snowflakes blow or have had to contend with
muddy, rutted roads while dust blows in the fields. Those are
experiences that, at the time, do not seem dissonant.

Keeping an eye on the weather was not just a pastime for us,
it was survival. Last night I watched the weather report to see
what I would face on my drives this week. I got a report for
the whole week, and I can depend on it to be reasonably
accurate. As a child, weather reports were several days old
before we got them. So we kept an eye on the clouds. Many
conversations were interrupted because someone got up and
went outside to look at the sky.

There were rules to follow. When my Father was a boy, he
knew to bring the team of horses in if it looked stormy. Likewise, when John was a boy, he knew to bring the tractor in
from the field if there were storm clouds. If a cool breeze

came in when it had been hot, we knew hail was coming. And during the cool-down time of a hot day, Daddy would stand on the porch, watching for tornado clouds in the southwest.

When Daddy had retired from farming to Hope, he would ask, without fail, when we drove up from Wichita, "What does the wheat look like down there?" or "Have you had any rain?" It was not idle talk. That was survival for Kansas farmers. "If we get rain, we will be okay."

When Daddy was a child, his mother would say to him, "Dan, go get some fish for supper." And he would go out and get fish for supper. There was no question on her part, nor in his mind, as to what they would have for supper. The fish were there—he simply had to catch them. But before he died in 1979 my Father was worried that those same streams had dried up. He would often talk of how, when he was a child on the Brunner farm, water would gush up out of the mouth of the well pump after a heavy rain. That same well is now dry because the water level has fallen so low.

There has always been water on the prairie but not always on *top* of the prairie. One day when I was a child, my Father showed me a place along the roadside a few hundred feet from our mailbox. There was an opening in it as big around as a coffee can, through which you could hear water. Daddy dropped a stone into it, and it was a long time before it hit water. I imagine it was somehow connected to the Huenquenet Cave, which was located about a half mile from the corner of our farm.

The entrance to the Huenquenet had been filled in by the farmer who owned the property and did not want his cattle falling into it. When I was in high school, people came to excavate the cave. They had read the reports of bags of gold hidden there by bandits who had robbed a carrier on the Santa Fe Trail on the early frontier. Supposedly, the gold was hidden in the Huenquenet because it was not far from the Santa Fe Trail. It has never been recovered, and there is nothing to prove that it was actually there. But as long as there is a suspicion of gold, there will always be adventurers who come to find it.

On a nice day in Washington, D.C., last winter, I tried to explain Kansas weather to a cab driver. It was January, and we were discussing the light snow that had fallen. I told him about a bad "white-out" (wind blowing snow so hard that even a small amount of snow makes vision impossible) on the western Kansas plains. When I told him that a school bus driver once got lost in a white-out, the cab driver shrugged his shoulders and asked, "Why didn't he just follow the street?"

A blizzard is dangerous. Like many farmers in the 1950s, my Father augmented our farm income as a road patrolman for the county, and he was out in the very worst of weather. One night the huge road maintainer got stuck in a drift and Daddy walked home. He almost didn't make it. At one point, he crawled into a snow bank and began dozing off to sleep. Rousing himself, he crawled over high piles of snow until he finally made it home. As he sat before the stove, thawing his fingers in cold water, I saw my Father cry. I had never seen him cry from pain before. Even the tips of his ears were frozen.

It has been a long time since Grandpa was our weatherman and Daddy went outside "to check the clouds." High-tech Doppler systems now provide warnings when Kansas communities are threatened by tornadoes. But we still shrug our shoulders, look at each other, and say "That's Kansas. You don't like the weather, just wait a while."

Mother has been moaning. In an effort to change her focus, I decide to sing a hymn. I say, "Mother, Mother, I'm going to sing." She opens her eyes and looks at me. "Well, everyone's been warned."

Nurses check on her often now. She is becoming too hard for me to handle. Helen picks her up like she is a baby, and I marvel at her strength and tenderness. Most people really do not understand what nurses of geriatric patients go through, day after day, patient after patient. If they did, nurses would be some of the highest-salaried people in our nation.

Now, in spite of our differences of opinion about how to treat Mother as she dies, and with the exception of the feeding frenzy, I know this little hospital is giving Mother excellent physical care.

Today Helen has difficulty getting Mother back into bed and I start giggling. Then we both get to laughing and Helen can't do anything but lean against the bed, hold Mother, and laugh. Aunt Dixie is there and she starts laughing, too. "Mother," I assure her, "we're laughing at Helen, not you."

One nurse we affectionately call Sarge. She is stocky and

brusque and very capable. At first Mother was frightened of the Sarge, but she has made peace with her, and now she looks forward to seeing her come in. This nurse talks to her as if Mother were a lady in her parlor whom Sarge had come to visit, not somebody lying on her back in a hospital. "Alice," she'll say, "guess what I did today?" She doesn't censor her conversation, and it is good for Mother. Things are lighter, more normal when Sarge is around.

Helen decides to take Mother for a stroll, which is no easy thing with the IV pole. But we make it down to the waiting room farthest from the skilled nursing unit. We sit and talk for a while, joking with a few people who pass by. Mother, once so alert to everything, ignores them. Even so, Helen believes it is good for Mother to get away from her room. A nurse/friend from Hope sticks her head in the door and says, "There you are! I've been looking for you." She pushes the lock-out button on the morphine. It gives Helen an idea, and she fabricates a story she wants told to Sarge.

So the nurse dutifully goes back to the desk and reports she found the saline solution on a pole by the curb, the morphine gone, and a white van like Helen's disappearing around the corner. Sarge hollers, "What?" Exactly what Helen wanted. As we return past the nurses' station, Sarge looks up and yells at us. It is good to laugh.

Coming back through the prairie at twilight, I see the blue-stem grass and the broomweed changing color as the light moves down in the sky. Before I get back to Topeka it is dark. The night weaves its magic. Everything is close together. Lights that look to be just over the hill are actually many miles away. Illusions abound on the prairie and in the room where Mother is dying. Our reality is a distortion of time and distance, both physically and mentally, and I am alone on the prairie with my thoughts.

August 17

"Come back into my heart.
I need your love. I need your care."

Today Mother is oblivious to anyone around her. In the midst
of praying, "Come back into my heart, I need your love, I
need your care," she turns sharply toward the door as though
hearing someone speak. "Heavenly Father?" she asks, listening. Urgently, and a little louder, "Heavenly Father?" Then
sharply, "Heavenly Father?" I want to know what she is hearing, but I do not intrude.

In the middle of the afternoon she wakes from a sleep and
murmurs, "I just hope . . . I just hope He keeps me safe."
"Mother," I say, "that's a promise!" She is quiet, then whispers "promise . . . chapter." She is trying to sing a little song
she sang as a child in Sunday School. "Every promise in the
Book is mine; every chapter, every verse, every line." She
mouths the words while I sing it for her. She lies quietly for a
while and then says "Precious Lord." It is one of her favorites.
"Precious Lord, take my hand. Lead me on, help me stand.
I am tired, I am weak, I am worn . . ."

I have learned my capacity for caffeine. I know two cups of
coffee will keep me awake for six hours. On trips to and from

the hospital, I use caffeine to keep me alert. I leave the hospital on this evening, alert but saddened, feeling a deep sense of loss and wonderment.

I look at the darkened hills, remembering my heritage and the "taming" of this land: the people who left England and Sweden, the Germans from Russia who came here and made farmland out of the prairie. Now there is talk of making a national park in the Flint Hills for the purpose of preserving the prairie and turning some acreage back to grasslands. Donavon says the farmers are now in the same situation Plains Indians faced when this land was taken from them by the settlers. An interesting thought.

I've heard it said that less than one percent of the tall-grass prairie that once grew in the heart of America is still here. And it occurs to me that must be what we mean by "endangered." Twice endangered. Extinction or neon lights and QuikTrips that would rim a prairie park would change the grasslands forever. It is far too fragile for such phony intrusions.

The grass grows on a thin layer of topsoil over rock. It is so thin there are parts of Kansas where one can still find ruts from the hundreds of iron-bound wooden wheels of heavily laden wagons following the trails west 150 years ago. Today, dirt bikers are clamoring for ranchers to open up huge acreages for their pleasure, and the land is continually at risk from the Big Red One. Fort Riley, in all its military splendor, has encroached into the grasslands. Imagine caterpillar tanks driven across the thin layer of soil where little else but grass can grow. If the topsoil goes, the grass goes. With intrusions of buildings and fences, expanse and distance disappear. One quick decision on the part of government and the Flint Hills ecosystem could change forever.

These thoughts, like my Mother's impending death, haunt me. I want the Flint Hills to be here after we are gone. It is a land both simple and complex. On the surface it looks plain and safe, but you have to be aware of the unfamiliar in order to survive. You have to know where to look for water. The direction that grass bends is important to safe passage in a storm. And you have to understand the cloud formations, for they can boil into dangerous storms or roil into a tornado.

I do not "own" any of this land, yet it is mine as surely as if I held the deeds to thousands of acres. Several of my cousins have large acreages, but what is theirs is mine, for I h 'e learned to capture it with my eyes and with my heart. All I have to do is look at it, be surrounded by it, and it is mine, again.

Culture . . . in Mother's violin and Elmer's musical saw,
Clara's poems and Eva's songs, dances at Pilsen and
Brethren foot-washing rituals.

I am at home today, trying to store up energy for trips to the
hospital. So I have been reading all afternoon and just finished
another book about Kansas settlers. I am disappointed again.
I wish it had been written by an easterner, but it wasn't. This
was a Kansan implying that the early settlers were uneducat-
ed and uncultured.

The men and women who first broke the sod of the prairie
were often the first Europeans to walk the lands they plowed.
And they were fiercely proud of how they survived. Today, it
is their original homesteads, broken down, unpainted, decay-
ing, that lie like tarnished medals around the neck of the
Flint Hills.

134   My Father's people, the Germans from Russia, sought to
firmly establish their culture, to use it freely. It was not to be.
It could not be for more than a generation. A sky and a land
that bare the soul are instruments for change. So they adapted.
Where they came from and who their parents were probably
had less to do with who I am than the tall-grass prairie on
which they chose to reside.

Both my Father's and my Mother's ancestors were people who thrived on the quiet, still life, who appreciated and respected the land on which they worked. At first, they farmed the new land with familiar ways brought from the Old Country. As land-grant colleges and "specialists" sprang up, some farmers began to modify farming practices. Still some of them resisted. Electric lines hooked up to Grandfather's barn allowed him to use machines he'd never before used. County agents told him how to get the most out of his land. That those agents were partly wrong was something we would not know for a long time.

My grandparents worked hard and despised laziness. They had to haul supplies a long way, so they became adept at fixing and inventing. They were independent, but also dependent upon neighbors. They would do anything for a neighbor and expected that neighbor to do the same for them. If the neighbor failed when he was needed, that didn't keep my grandparents from helping him the next time he called (it was done with a martyr's air), but there wouldn't be a soul in the county who didn't know that the neighbor had not responded in time of need. And in a land where you were expected to "make do" against any and all odds, the man who let his wife and children go hungry or without clothing was a man scorned by the community as "no good." "Just plain no good" was the worst epithet my parents ever used.

The culture of the early settlers was in transition, but it was there. My Father's culture was manifested in two languages, English and German.

Just as culture was there in southeastern Kansas when Mrs. English stored her grand piano on its side in a sod dugout and carried it outside to be played, culture was also there in Mother's violin and Elmer's musical saw, in Eva's songs and in Clara's poems. Culture was there in the myriad books and magazines that farm folk read and traded and cherished. Culture was there in the prairie flower fresh each morning on the table and in the bierocks served on that table at noon. (Bierocks, bread rolls with cabbage and meat baked in them, come from a blending of two cultures—Russian and German.) Culture was there in the all-night dances at Ramona, Pilsen, and Tampa. Culture was there in the fancy dresses made out of flour sacks, in the little bonnets and long black dresses of the Amish, and in Harriet's quilts. It was there whenever the River Brethren held foot-washing ceremonies, the Lutherans worshiped in German, the Baptists knelt at tent meeting, and the Catholics held a wake.

Early settlers knew that survival was more than food to eat or a roof over their heads. But culture on the prairie was not something they went to see someone else perform for an hour a week. The cultured life of the prairie people was much different than that on the coasts. No better or worse, just different.

August 21

I've been talking to her sister on the phone. I ask, "Mother, do you want to say goodbye to Aunt Helen?" She says, "I'd rather say hello."

I leave my mother at 8:15 tonight and the sunset is purple. I pray, "Father, don't let her suffer. If you can, take her tonight, and if you don't, please let her feel calm."

Sometimes at the hospital, I silently pray, "Take her now, please," and aloud, "Father, take care of your servant Alice on this journey. Let her feel our love go with her as we know hers will always be with us." She answers, "Amen."

I really thought today was her last day with us. Her hands were blood-red hot, and her eyes rolled back in her head. She would often stop breathing, and one time I counted up to fourteen slowly before she took another breath. I am concerned that she has no pain relief. At five, I asked at the desk for an RN. "I'm an LPN." I walked the entire hospital and couldn't find a registered nurse. They were eating, I guess. And those on the floor were too busy to sit at the desk. I have sympathy for them. They are overworked and underpaid. But I still needed help.

I felt desperate, alone, fearful for my Mother's care, and absolutely horrified at some of the things being done to her body now that she can no longer say "no." The veins in her arms have collapsed, and the doctor has put a plate in her chest in order to use the vein in her neck.

The morphine drip had been stopped the night before, then increased this morning. Apparently they were concerned about her breathing. The apnea worried me, too. I sat on the edge of her bed for a long time today to let her feel my closeness.

But on the way home, my hands double into fists on the steering wheel and a scream builds up within me, threatening to overpower me. Nursing this feeling, I come up out of the craggy Geary County bluffs and I see the hills ending in the sky. I am instantly subdued, and the knowledge that this is the biggest thing I know, bigger than my anger, bigger than my fear, comes again. My big sky will always be here. The physical world lets my fear subside, and I know once again I do not have to be in control of this thing called death. It is not within my ability to do so. I am a part of this time and this place but not the master of it. What is happening is supposed to happen. And if it isn't, then it is not my "goof-up." I do not have to fix it or change it. I am only a some-time traveler on this prairie.

August 25

Today Mother talks about her impending death.
"It's coming so soon," she says.

Mother is agitated, so I sing along with the recording of
hymns I had made in June for her. She listens, then turns to
me and says, "It's soon time to go to sleep." She won't say die.

In the afternoon she begins a litany, "I hurt, I hurt, I hurt."
She has apnea for ten to twenty-two seconds. I hear her say,
"She goes into my heart every time I go to sleep." Later on,
during pain, she says, "I must put in an order . . ." Finally a
nurse comes in and gives Mother more medicine.

I worry about her and I am curious. I ask, "Can you see me,
Mother?" "Oh, yes. . . . Can you wait until Jesus comes?"
Again I sing to her to try to stop the moaning. She sometimes repeats the phrases, trying to sing with me. I know
today she is comforted by the hymns.

Suddenly an aide comes in and slams the door shut. I believe
she did not want to hear me sing.

"Let's get her up."
"Why?" I ask.

"Because she needs to be up."

"For how long?"

"Oh, just a short period."

She goes after another nurse, since it is obvious I am not going to help. In frustration I go out for a cup of coffee. When I come back thirty minutes later, Mother lies slung back in the chair, her head thrown back, unable to hold it up. "Oh, I want to lay down." I call for the aide and ask that Mother be put back in bed. Now she is in so much pain they have to increase the dosage. I know there is a fine line between letting her deteriorate by lying there and keeping her mobile so she will be more comfortable. But it is obvious getting her up wears her out, and I feel they should not be doing that now.

On the way home I relive the events of the day. Everything I believe about dying is being cast aside while my Mother dies. There is nothing "whole" here. They see only a body, a body that was important when it could be repaired. Now, when it cannot be "fixed," they do a few things to Band-Aid her body while ignoring her "self," which is still strong inside.

Hopefully, the medical attendants are not aware of what they do. But perhaps they are aware. When Donavon had a heart attack in the summer of 1990, his surgeon said to him, "I am a mechanic. I take care of the mechanical part of your heart." Very "up-front." There was Donavon, trying to become his own body's caretaker, and the surgeon did not want to deal with anything beyond the "mechanical."

And now Mother has an excellent surgeon, who takes care of those parts of her body on which he can make improvements. But he has left her spirit all alone to cope with the dying of the shell in which she has lived for almost eighty years.

Can she do it? In spite of the separation, can she pull it off? The answer is in the wind past my car. A windstorm troubling the grass on the prairie (with no one to see) still blows. Mother's spirit living in a dying body (with no one to see) still moves.

August 27

> John leans over and asks, "Mother is there anything
> I can do for you?"
> "Just be a good boy, John."

John and Maggie have been coming to the hospital nightly.
Mother looks forward to it. She has never wanted us to call
Margaret by the name "Maggie," even though we all do. In
front of Mother we try to say Margaret but sometimes we
slip, laugh, and now we have started calling her Maggie Margaret to cover all bases.

Today, under the influence of the morphine, Mother is confused about time. The events of our childhood are coming
back to her. This doesn't happen often. Last week, though,
John said she had been sleeping and when she awoke, she
raised her head and said, "John! John! You are going to spill
your milk!"

Tonight as he gets ready to leave, he bends down to kiss her
and asks, "Is there anything I can do for you?" She murmurs,
"Just be a good boy, John." He tells me about it in our late
night phone conversation. "That's what she used to tell me
when I was a kid," he says. I hang up the phone and true to
my heritage, write down my thoughts:

He was just a little boy on a struggling Kansas farm, throwing his ball and letting his dog fetch it. Then, growing tired and hungry, he tugged at the tail until doggy yelped. From the kitchen window came the call he always knew would come,

"Be a good boy, John."

He was an ordinary prairie kid getting up at dawn to feed the chickens first, then eat his oatmeal and toast. Books, coat, cap . . . bus waiting down the lane. And always, Mom standing at the door, dinner pail in hand, and a pat for his back.

"Be a good boy, John."

Graduating from Rural High, attending college down the way, then joining the Marines, her first child to leave home. Suitcase in hand, he turns his back on the country kitchen with its forever-to-be-remembered smells. The goodbyes are said, the car door shut, she stands in the yard with eyes full of tears.

"Be a good boy, John."

He makes a handsome groom, this man full grown who loves a woman with three fatherless children to raise. He brings them home to his mother who blesses his instant family, letting them stay there until they get their feet on the ground. Then he leaves her house for the last time and her eyes follow them down the road.

"Be a good boy, John."

Middle-aged and busy with his job, he visits the hospital night-ly on this vigil at his Mother's death. He says loudly (for her hearing is poor), "Mom, is there anything you need?" Her eyes are closed as he stoops to give that last kiss, and he hears her whisper, one last time, those words from long ago,

"Just be a good boy, John."

August 28

A Dance with Death

Today she is not able to talk. I am sad for her and I am sad
for me. Her transition, from this life to the next, has become
a nightmare. I begin to wonder if the inability of others to
discuss her dying is creating doubts and fears for her. It feels
as if I, who would have her live forever, am alone in saying,
"She's dying, see how she dies." The response is always,
"She's living, see how she lives."

We are participating in an awkward, whirling, driven dance
with pain controlling each beat. A dose of morphine and the
song becomes a dirge. We are in slow motion. She languish-
es. Her breathing is nearly gone.

> Pain and ease, pain and ease.
> Round and round, so pretty please,
> "Save her now!" "No, let her go!"
> Fast and gay, sad and slow.

The pain belongs to her, the ease to them. Her dying is at the
pleasure of someone else. I am confused by her reality and
their arrogance. And in my mind the thoughts scramble:

> Hot is cold, cold is hot.
> Here is pain, pain is not.

So I hold her tight, tell her goodbye a thousand times. She wants to die. We are both ready. Then swiftly the dance changes.

A nurse brings more food, gives another shot. In the silent room my heart screams, "Leave her alone. See, she dies." Though she has her white-clothed back to me and is busy with my mother, I feel, rather than hear, the age-honored response her profession has embraced. "She's living! See how she lives."

"Let her go," I wordlessly cry. Now borne on the impulses of air in this feeling-charged room comes the unspoken answer, "We can't do that." I weep alone. "I'm sorry, Mother, I thought it was your day to die."

I leave the hospital. Not wanting to be alone with my thoughts, I turn on the radio. In Wichita, ninety miles away, the abortion conflict rends the city apart. Outsiders have come to Kansas to "teach a reverence for life." They let hate fill their hearts in order to make a singular point about when life begins. We really are hung up on when life begins and when it ends. Driving along I-70 and listening to the news coverage, I realize that if these folks believe life begins with conception and ends with death, then they don't believe their own religious teachings. They are prolife, they say. And they talk of the right to life. A right to life? If you have a right to life, then don't you have a right to the strongest, healthiest, wisest life? No one has a right to life. Life simply is. And one day it isn't.

And now my thoughts come fast, with the shouts of arrogance on the radio background. A respect for living means a respect for dying because things living have to die so other things might live. And when people lay down their lives for others in war or in some other selfless act, we honor them and give them medals.

In the animal world, in order to live, something else must die. When native people of the plains had to kill bison for food, they used a ceremony that included an apology for the killing and a thank you for sustaining life. Everything living feeds on something dead or dying. Death is important to life. To accept life, I must accept death.

The radio intrudes. I turn it off and watch the prairie flow by. A clear horizon ahead, sky and grass and wind now whisper me my song, "Mother is dying! Mother is dying!" A response comes on the wind rushing past the car, pushing this year's dying grass in waves . . . "Everything dies! Everyone dies!"

Around a curve and pointed east, the wind comes back with renewed vigor. My thoughts are a roar in my head. "Mother is dying, I will die, so will my children and one day, my grand-children." As my thoughts pulsate, the wind breaks over me again and again and finally calms. My thoughts become a gentle whisper. I see, alongside the road and up on the hills, dead grass. Near the watering holes, grasses are sagging toward decomposition. Going down, down, into the labyrinth of roots. There, unseen, the roots will feed in the nutrient-rich soil until one day, in the spring of a new year, blades begin their upward climb toward the sun. Yes! Born anew some fine prairie morning. The words feel right on the wind. I am okay within.

August 31

"I only want to go to sleep."

They have discontinued the breathing treatments, which she
fought. During the last two months, whenever the therapist
left the room, I would take the mask and hold it back away
from her face. I know the treatment didn't do her as much
good, but she wasn't so terrified then. I could hardly stand
to see her struggling against the mask. Usually I just left the
room because I knew it was the right thing for her. Her doctor paid careful attention to certain things; one of them was
breathing therapy. Choking was what she had always feared.
Today, they tell me the doctor discontinued the treatments. I
wonder if the nurses think I complained. This time I am not
guilty.

One of our favorite nurses was there today. I told her I heard
that mother had a bad night with no sleep. She said she had
arrived at 4 A.M. and the door was closed. "I don't like that,"
the nurse said. Before I left, I talked to nurses at both desks
about leaving Mother's door open in case she needs someone in the night.

In the midst of her moaning Mother says, "I've never seen it
so nice." Later, she says, "I want to go home, I want to go
home, Mama said . . ." and I cannot hear the rest. Half an
hour later she rallies and begins to call her sisters' names,

"Helen, Edna, Helen, Edna, Helen, Edna." "She wanted to come back and see me before." (I believe this refers to Helen, who lives in Illinois.) "She wanted to go as much as I did." (I believe this means Edna, who is in a nursing home.) And then, with resignation, she murmurs, "I only want to go to sleep."

Aunt Helen calls and I tell her about Mother's condition. I ask her if she wants to talk to Mother and she says, "No, if it hasn't been said by now, it isn't there to say." She goes on to talk about the relationship they had, saying that they were there for each other whenever they were in need. "I certainly don't need to run over at the last minute," she said. "The loving and caring has been all along." Oh, how true that is.

Aunt Helen is a nurse, as is my sister Helen. There has been a nurse in the last three generations of our family. Great Aunt Edith was head nurse at Fort Riley during its terrible flu epidemic and was honored by the Red Cross when she died. And then my Aunt Helen became a nurse. Now, Aunt Helen reminds me of when my Grandmother Clara had a stroke. She had been in the kitchen of their farm west of Hope. Grandpa had been lying on the dining room couch, and Grandma somehow managed to make it to him. He immediately got up and helped her lie down. She was not able to talk, but she did get him to understand she wanted a pencil and paper. So he brought them to her and she wrote,

"Helen will come." Helen was living six hundred miles away near Chicago, but she was the daughter Grandma wanted, for she was a nurse and Grandma could depend on her. "Helen" has been a household word for two generations in our family.

LIGHTNING

The lightning has come again to the prairie. Soon after comes the drum roll crescendo of thunder, and then the prairie orchestra begins its symphony in earnest. There is the pop of lightning streaking through the sky. The answer of thunder is sometimes loud and banging. At other times, it begins slow and far away, rumbling to an audience on the eastern side of this prairie theater. Building and backing away. Building again. Now backing away. How I love those low far-away rumbles. They lull you. Don't be fooled. Now! A clap of thunder boxes your ears. Prairie kids are often told, "The thunder won't hurt you. Be glad for the thunder. If you hear it, you know that the lightning didn't strike you!"

Now the lightning exerts itself. Prima donna–like, it demands your utmost attention. It lights up the darkness and plays "catch me if you can" across the broad expanse of sky. Sometimes it strikes at some unseen alien in the air and at other times, it streaks up the dome to disappear in wondrous clouds of color. Thunder! Lightning! Wonder! Fear! Excitement! The tall-grass hills are magnificent in a lightning storm. And when it is over, you are hollow inside, clean as the new washed prairie, and ready . . .

ON THE
PRE-AGRARIAN
PRAIRIE

Last Scene

There is a pulsation beneath the burnt stubble. Roots, under stress, begin to multiply and grow even as the first raindrops fall. A distant thunder. Rain spatters the scorched earth. In seconds, the wind is pushing sheets of water down the prairie's yawning cracks. As parched grasses soak up the rain, rivulets fill dry creek beds.

Tomorrow, sun and wind will again play on the prairie. New grass will grow. Hundreds of prairie flowers will bloom. The bison will return. But today, prairie animals scurry to find shelter on high ground. The old and those weakened from yesterday's fire now fall beneath the relentless rain. Only the strong survive on the prairie.

FROM THE DIARY
IN SEPTEMBER

September 1

> Go south of Hope on a county road until you are a mile
> north of Marion/Dickinson county line. At the Rosebank
> church, turn west onto a dirt road that runs south of the
> graveyard. Go 3/4 mile to a prairie lane on the north side
> of the road, 1/4 mile long. Not passable in wet weather.

No one has been here for a long time. Grass has grown over
the lane I walked as a child and a fence has been strung across
it. But a few feet beyond, I see the farmer's gate. I stop the
car, open the gate, and drive through. Closing the gate behind
me, I proceed on a difficult course, following the farmer's
tractor path down the pasture toward my old homestead.
The car bucks and surges on the rough trail. It is obvious the
path is used only when the farmer returns to care for his cattle.

This is the place where I first saw the wind. I was eight years
old when I became aware that wind is visible on the grasslands.
Grasses bend as great airflows roll over them. I would lie in
those same grasses and watch the motion above. I am so
sorry for people who have never done that.

Now I stand where I once played in the sun and wind. The
house is gone, only the foundation remains. The barn is gone.

Of my childhood home, only the windmill and the stock tank are left. There are no fences. Cattle have free range.

I walk beneath the aged apricot trees in the shelter belt, searching for my old playhouse. But only the trees and the tall grass wait for me in this quiet place. The grasses are a far more fitting memorial for my Father than the cold stone in the cemetery five miles north.

I walk south, seeking old landmarks. Here is where the garden was, here the old granary, here the milk house, here the tree that pushed at my window on windy nights, and here the front gate. "Please do not swing on the gate, Carol."

My parents did not become wealthy from the farmland, but they were good caretakers of the soil. I search for some memento to take back with me and then I find, hidden in the tall grass, a four-foot length of crooked Osage orange, the corner post of our yard. It is weathered, full of holes, and the wood has been polished where cattle have rubbed against it. I carefully put it into the car.

I drive back through the bumpy pasture and I feel good. Today I went home and found that the prairie had reclaimed my childhood home.

September 4

"Who all came?"

"Just me . . . just Carol."

"Is that the only one they could get rid of?"

I stand there looking down at her. Her eyes are closed and she has a feeble grin on her face. She now weighs less than a hundred pounds, and I think what a giant of a woman this is. I silently pray, "Thank you, thank you, thank you for this Mother who taught us to laugh at life."

I look more attentively at her, wondering how long this can continue. It is obvious her body is wearing out. Her legs lie so still and mold into a flat position when she is not moved for a time. Now I see her eyes are open. Mother is watching me watch her. She looks at me very closely and asks, "Do the little bones in your legs crack sometimes when you move them?" It catches me by surprise and I begin to cry. I cannot answer. She does not need an answer. She just wants me to know she knows her body is deteriorating. I reach over and hold her and it is quiet in the room.

I can see wind blowing trees outside the hospital window. It is blowing harder than usual today. My nemesis and my comforter, this Kansas wind. Thirty years ago when we moved to the heart of Indianapolis for a three-year stay, the thing I missed most was Kansas wind. One night the wind came up and I didn't get to bed all night. I just listened. With the window open and the curtains blowing, the wind took me home again to Kansas. Ah, Hoosiers, you didn't know for whom the wind blew one night.

The winds of my childhood . . . warm breezes pushing the curtain against my bed, strong winds letting me sleep to dream. When the wind came up and it was storming, Daddy would stand out on the porch braced against the wind, watching to the southwest for a tornado. He was our early warning system. I loved the wind so much as I grew older, I never minded going to school windblown. There were girls in those days of bouffant hair styles who ducked away from the wind, whining about its effects on their hair. I never noticed because the wind was my companion always and my comforter frequently. The sound of a good strong wind can still put me to sleep at night.

Now I glance out the window. The sky looks ominous and I am glad Mother doesn't see it. When I go out in the hall, one of the nurses says tornadoes have been sighted south of us. It is time to go. I start home under a sky full of threatening clouds.

I speed north hoping to outrun the weather behind me. By the time I turn east at the junction of the Smoky Hill and Republican rivers, the sky is clear over me, but on the horizon there are clouds and a brilliant lightning storm about fifty miles away, somewhere near Topeka. I feel a sense of loss that I am missing it mixed with a sense of security because it isn't happening to me and just a tinge of fear since I am moving toward it. My nerves are on edge, my adrenaline heightened.

Stories handed down from my greatgrandparents Robinson tell of lightning flashing around the iron-bound wheels of the covered wagon on their first trip across the prairie. And I can imagine the fear and utter helplessness of my Greatgrand-mother as she shrank under the canvas cover.

It is still a singular feeling to be caught in a storm on the open prairie. Now the West has been tilled, there are no "fireballs" on the ground as in Greatgrandma's time. But I know, as she did, that the storm will soon be over, marching on to some other theater and some other audience.

When I reach home in the evening I get a phone call from Lance. The good-news/bad-news rocks me. The good news has to do with Granddaughter Kasia's writing talent. I am glad she is going to school in the city that was the home of William Allen White, one of the most beloved and respected newspapermen in Kansas history. I am proud. Then Lance tells me his wife M'Liz is being tested and may be ill. "I'm okay," she insists. I get off the phone and I wonder what else can come into my life. I need it to stop. Things are going too fast. Can't I finish Mother's dying first?

September 6

I am remembering a day when I was fourteen. It was nearly noon, and I was still curled up in bed while the women of my family toiled over boilers in the backyard. Mother understood. She made excuses for me, "Carol is busy. She has to practice," she said.

There had been activity in the barnyard since sunup. The big kettles were moved to the back porch. The sausage stuffer was borrowed from Uncle Alex. Daddy took the gun outside. I went upstairs and pulled the covers over my head. I shut out the sights and sounds, but I couldn't quit thinking about butchering. I was sick to my stomach. I hated those days.

In a family where you do the unpleasant when survival depends on it, it was not acceptable to be squeamish about food preparation. I did get so I could clean chickens by not thinking of them as the chicks that followed me around the yard. But I never could chop off their heads or be around when Aunt Gay swung them back and forth to snap off their heads. Because Mother so completely understood my problem, I thought she must have felt the same way. It would have been typical for her not to let anyone know, those forty years ago.

During the past year and a half, while Mother lived alone, the tables were reversed. I helped her with her fear that she would die in the night and not be found by calling her every morning at 7:30. "Hello," I'd hear her quavering voice. It was obvious she had spent the early morning hours pacing the floor. I tried to be cheerful and was careful not to tell her too much about what Donavon and I had in our busy schedules because it only served to point out her own perceived idleness.

So I would talk to her about the prairie we both loved. "Remember how in the fall, cottonwood trees lose leaves from the bottom up, until at winter, all that is left is a crown of leaves across the uppermost branches? Did you ever notice that from a distance, they look like thousands of little prairie birds perched on top?"

"Oh yes they do," she says delightedly.

Or I'd tell her about things I'd read. "I saw a diary kept by a sixteen-year-old girl who, with her family, were the first Europeans to the Solomon area. She recorded over one hundred flowers on the pristine prairie from May to August that first year."

163

"Yes," Mother says, and for a moment her memory intercedes on her behalf, "the flowers of the prairie are special. Some people call them weeds." We laugh together.

September 7

Some things I have learned.

I am cleaning house today. It is getting quite clean. Joel once told me he remembered from his childhood that when I was upset I would clean house. The night my mother-in-law died I went home at 2 A.M. and got down on my hands and knees to mop the kitchen floor. Even my neighbors have known my propensity for work when upset. One day I was in the yard furiously tackling the weeds in the bed of vines on the north side of our house when I heard Margaret, my next door neighbor remark, "You and Don must have had quite a fight!"

It was my Mother who showed me how to get busy when things went wrong. I have only recently realized how valuable a thing she taught me. She also understood the importance of doing nothing.

Nothing was something I sometimes did as a child. I would lie on my back in the pasture watching the clouds over me and the planes winging Wichita-way. It is possible to spend an entire afternoon doing that while waiting for the Schimming kids to come over for a ballgame in the pasture. Sometimes I followed the little rills made by waterways down cattle paths, and even when the waterways were dry I was fascinated by them.

In my mind I can see the corral where the salt block stands, a beautiful creation by those low-lifes of the prairie as their tongues swirl around and around, carving their statue. I bend down and taste it, too. Up toward the barn, the well is pumping. Water is gushing into the stock tank with its load of water lilies pushed over away from where the cattle drink. Daddy has put some bullhead catfish in the tank and they have grown large. Up on the windmill step about six feet high is the old cup Daddy used to get a drink. He left it there the day he moved from the farm, when he got his last cold drink, hung it up, and walked away.

I mentally climb through the bars on the big gate, and on one side is the garden where I spent many a late-summer day, hunkered down on the ground beside the tomato vines with the kitchen saltshaker, sampling the most delightful of all tastes—a warm ripe tomato. I must quick get the salt-shaker back to the kitchen before Mother sees it is gone!

North of the windmill is the barn, weathered and now moved several inches on its foundation from a tornado one spring. In the little milk house is the cream separator I washed day after day. Over eighty disks (skimming chambers) had to be separated and cleaned. From that chore of my youth, I learned I was responsible and that I had to do the tedious: to keep going until it was done. I hated washing the separator, but Mother had drilled into me how important cleanliness was to our health and our ability to sell the cream. It wasn't until decades later I figured out how the old cream separator helped make me who I am. A woman who now scrubs the floor, the tub, the sink, and the stove until she scrubs away her frustration and her fear.

September 9

"See you in the morning, Mother!"

What a day. She didn't talk, just looked at us. She looked and looked with such overwhelming love in her eyes. She looked as though she was trying to memorize every line in our faces.

She has been force-fed by spoon all along. Today, an aide comes in with a tray, puts it down and looks at Mother, then says to Helen and me, "You do what you want with that." I am so grateful for her understanding.

I meet with the hospital administrator today and we talk over Mother's financial situation. Then I start talking about the large amounts of food she is getting. He says, "We're not going to starve her to death." Around and around we go. "Listen," I say, "you don't take a woman who has eaten only a bowl of soup and a few crackers for supper the last two years and now suddenly stuff her with a full dinner! All that does is exacerbate her hiatal hernia." I try medical rather than moral arguments, and we find some common ground. He says we can meet with the nurses at a staffing.

I am in conflict about her care. On one hand, I believe the hospital is prolonging Mother's death unnecessarily and her well-being and dignity are secondary to the protection of someone else's standards and someone else's fear of death. But on the other hand, some of the measures they use certainly do help ease her dying.

Mother has never been afraid of death, just of dying. And now the hospital staff is unwilling to dignify her life by accepting her dying. It is as if she is on a journey and everyone refuses to recognize her destination. This makes her trip meander through a maze of confusion.

There are deep misunderstandings. John, Helen, and I deal with this in our own ways, but we are of one accord in these areas: Mother knew she was dying when she entered the hospital, she wanted her children around her during her last days, and she was anticipating an afterlife of joy. Yet any attempts to discuss her dying bring accusations of euthanasia—a subject that has absolutely nothing to do with our situation. As a consequence, what should be a time of anticipation for Mother and her children has resulted in long and lonely nights, uncertainties, and the neglect of our larger families.

Death in this room has become a deep, dark secret about which no one talks. I wish they would just view Mother's death as closure to a well-lived life. They could let her eat what is comfortable for her and give her the kind of medicines that are the easiest to get down. They could help her to be calm as she faces death by recognizing and treating *both* physical and mental stress. They could talk to her about what she is facing. They could say "I don't know" when they don't.

Instead, they pretend that if Alice is fed well, she will get up out of that bed and go home. Their pretense doesn't fit into this scientific world and the air is charged with confusion.

It no longer is difficult to realize how prolonging death can be a living hell, for it is happening to Mother. And it's going to happen to all of us. Unless we die a fast accidental death, we too will face the transition (which is named death) to another phase (whose name is not known). Is how it happens of concern to others? Is the prolonging of death something others think about? Do they even know it is something they will face? Is it possible our whole society can ignore such an important part of our lives?

And now I must say a silent goodbye to Mother, for I am going to Denver for a week. I have decided I should be with Don in case he needs me. I ask John and Helen not to tell Mother. I will be talking to them and to her by phone. I think if she knows I will be gone she might try to live until I return. I don't want anything to keep her from dying. I am so curious about her will to live. I think it must be that all her life she has been a survivor. She has had to be strong, and she has had to struggle. Now her body is failing her and the will to live has kicked in again.

When I leave Mother tonight, I am fully aware she may die while I'm gone. I repeat our childhood parting, "See you in the morning, Mother!" And through my tears, I see her nod. On the road home, I remember that Mother never said "Good-bye" when we parted. She only said "I love you." And she never said "Good-night" when we went to bed. She only said, "See you in the morning." At home, I write my thoughts:

> I will see you in the morning
> When this night has passed away.
> Some prairie morning bright and clear
> Will be our kind of day.
>
> With the rooster's crow at dawning
> Comes the clean, new, sparkling sun
> Going fast unto the noon hour,
> We won't sit much past one!
>
> In the warmth of Kansas sunlight
> Fluffy clouds parade so free.
> That's the kind of day we'll have then,
> Custom-made for you and me.
>
> When the rosy sky at sunset
> Flings its color on each hand,
> I'll meet you just beyond the trees—
> We'll walk our tall-grass land.

But tonight the prairie's empty,
All my thoughts now need re-forming.
So I'll just say it like we used to—
I will see you in the morning!

September 11

"To love is to remember and my heart remembers you."

We are traveling across Kansas toward Denver. I feel the anticipated pleasure that has been mine since I was a child and first discovered that travel brought new sights and new ideas. But this time, there is dissonance. I feel out of place and cannot erase from my mind thoughts of a little hospital back in the Flint Hills where Mother waits to die.

When we stop in Wakeeney, I reach in my purse for change and find a slip of paper Helen gave me two days ago. On it are the words, "To love is to remember and my heart remembers you." Helen found it in her purse and thinks Mother might have put it there before she went to the hospital.

Mother never stopped collecting poems and pasting them in scrapbooks. But the ones Mother liked the most, she kept tucked away in her Bible close to her sewing chair. One such poem was sent to her by a friend after Daddy died. The message was that if Mother became lonely, she was to whisper Daddy's name and he would come in all the wonderful memories they share. He would not be far away.

It is a long way to the state line. Donavon and I talk about the eclipse we saw at the beginning of summer. That night we had gone for a walk, looking up at the stars and keeping track of the moon. I was thinking about Mother's dying and wishing our daughter were not half a world away. Suddenly I had the feeling that Doni, too, was watching the eclipse. What time would it be happening in Berlin? I felt close to her then and I remember wondering, "When Mother dies, will she be any further away from me than Doni is now?"

About two weeks later, when I was talking to Doni Marie on the phone, I told her about feeling close to her the night of the eclipse. She said she, too, had been looking at the moon that night from her room in Berlin, and she, too, had felt close to me. Our reactions during this eclipse would have happened at different times, given the distance. I wonder now what it means in relationship to death. If we could remove the boundaries of time and distance, what would happen to the boundaries between living and dying?

What if there were no "time"? What if we took away seconds, minutes, hours, days, and months from our remembrance? We would still have life experiences left, but where and when? And now I am beginning to sound like Doni Marie who, one night when she was a little girl, lay in bed looking up at the moon and wondering, "Where was God standing when he created the heavens and the earth?"

Life asks so many questions, offers so few answers. But I have learned to beware of the people who have all the answers, who leave no room for mystery.

INTERLUDE

Colorado is a place located west of Kansas. Its hills are some-what taller than ours. As a matter of fact, they are very pretty. But there is an enormous upthrust of rocks just outside Denver. It is not good for your lungs to try to get over them and it is too far to go around them. We would never tolerate that in Kansas.

Some Kansans go to Colorado because it is hard "to ski Kansas." I think some actually go just because it feels so good to come home again. So, you might as well stay in Kansas, where it takes a lot of looking to see, where the sun gets mighty serious about its comings and its goings, where the tall grass waves a friendly hello and the folks either like you or they don't. Mostly, they like you.

On the whole, I prefer Kansas.

174

September 18

    Keeping priorities in order.

Donavon and I are traveling I-70 on our way home from
Denver. He is sleeping, and I have been driving since we got
to the Kansas line. It is four hundred miles across Kansas, and
we have most of the distance to go. We travel the western
flatlands, mid-Kansas post rock country, and as we reach the
Flint Hills, sail on past the turnoff to Hope. Donavon needs
to get back to work this afternoon and we must keep on
going, but it is hard not to turn off. What is happening there?
Oh, so close to not turn down that way. Now we fly across
the breadth of the purple hills and continue toward timbered
eastern Kansas.

The wind is up and my hands grip the steering wheel. I know
the car is eating up gasoline trying to maintain speed against
this unseen assailant. I pass a stretch of land in Wabaunsee
County and see stripped trees outlined against the sky. They
were ravaged by the tornadoes of 1990, the year Helen's
house was destroyed. The tops of some of these trees are
gone. Many have twisted trunks that look like a giant hand
twirled them around and around the way you do spaghetti
on a fork. Some are lying at an angle, upended but still connected to the earth by their umbilical roots. Some will live
and some will not. It will take several years to realize the

total devastation of what journalist Howard Inglish has called the Year of the Storms.

Tornadoes are often seen on the prairie. Usually they come out of the Southwest. When their pattern differs, they are often more devastating. In May 1990, a tornado came out of the clouds from the northwest. A quarter-mile wide, it angled southeast across Marion County. A number of obstacles were in its way as it roared along the ground. These included a train, oil storage tanks in an oil field, silos, fences, telephone and light poles, and of course, animals, barns, and houses.

All these things, along with hundred-year-old trees, were sucked up into the stomach of the funnel, mixed with some acid of extreme malcontent, and then regurgitated back in a vile heap of vomit. One and a half miles west of Durham the tornado twisted the insides out of Tom and Helen's house and moved on, draping unrecognizable treasures over rock and pasture, leaving a Dali-like landscape in its wake.

Three hours after the tornado struck, we drove down the prairie through pitch-black night until we got to Helen's home, where some sixty Mennonite rescue workers were in the process of salvaging what was left of a lifetime. The glow of generated lights gave an eerie feeling to the already unreal scene. At 2 A.M. we went to a motel in McPherson to try to rest. At dawn we rose to make the necessary phone calls. We called Mother's brother Orville and asked him to tell Mother first that Helen and her family were all okay and then to tell her the house had been destroyed. We thought once Mother knew Helen was safe she wouldn't be too upset. And we were right. Not once did I hear Mother bemoan the loss of material goods. She just was grateful Helen's family had been saved. She accepted the tornado as she accepted everything else that life dealt her. Even when we drove her through the ravaged land to the home site, she just looked at it, and didn't say anything at all. She had her priorities in order.

Don and I get back to Topeka at noon. As soon as he leaves for work, I call Helen to see how Mother is. She doesn't tell me Mother is almost gone because she thinks I need to rest. "Don't come down today, come tomorrow like you had planned," Helen says. It gives me my "out." I am so very tired, and before I move from one world into another, I need to rest.

September 19

"Just an ordinary house on an ordinary piece of land."

Mother is weak and white. She doesn't eat and moans a lot.
She is aware of us and what we say. She will respond yes or
no. John says she has been "building a house" since I left.
"Just an ordinary house on an ordinary piece of land, so all
the kids will be home for Christmas." Tears come to my eyes.
There was so little room in the cottage in Hope and one day
we stopped having big family celebrations there. When the
family dinners were in her children's homes, Mother was
always the guest of honor and she never complained. But I
knew it wasn't like having us come home. And now as she lies
on her deathbed, we hear, for the first time, of her longing for
an ordinary house "so the kids will be home for Christmas."

The nurses have been wonderful. They come in and turn
her frequently and still get her up to go to the bathroom.
She sleeps a lot and is content to see Helen and me leave for
lunch. She doesn't seem to be in pain and continues to pray
out loud.

By evening I am trying to decide if I should stay all night, for
I know Helen will be gone tomorrow. She is going to Salina
for her continuing education credit. Finally Helen says, "Look,
I'll call Mother in the morning and if she is bad, I won't go to

Salina. You wait and come Saturday as you had planned." It is easy to agree for I am still tired out from our Colorado trip and I need to sleep in my own bed tonight.

The trip home is tough. Lingering in my brain is the thought that perhaps I should have stayed. Mentally I am under great stress, but I am so tired I refuse to think. I just turn on the cruise control and watch the road. I know its every bump and curve, and I follow the highway, my back and shoulder muscles knotted tightly against the world. I do not even watch the darkening hills. I am determined to not be comforted.

Miles go by. I'm not sure exactly where I am. It is difficult to tell where the sky begins and where earth ends, and since I haven't paid close attention, distance is meaningless. Now, as every night, the prairie has brought things near. I see lights and think the city is just a few miles away, when in reality it is more like fifteen.

I relax a little as I think about night trips north out of Wichita up the Kansas Turnpike, and how topping the last gentle rise, I see Emporia stretching along the horizon like a rhinestone necklace on a black velvet dress. I can travel and travel and the lights of Emporia are still spread out before me.

Now the night is dense black, and I want to reach out the

window and push aside the black curtain in front of my windshield. It is most oppressive. I know there is prairie around me, but I feel suspended in space. My senses are honed, open to this new experience. I am listening and waiting . . . what is it? What is happening to me? There is motion, something is changing. Of that I am sure. Is it on the prairie? Or is it in me?

September 20

Going home to Mother, one last time.

5 A.M.: Helen calls to tell me she checked with the hospital and Mother had a good night. When one of the nurses walked in earlier this morning, she said "How are you, Alice?" and Mother had looked so bright and cheerful and said "Well, how are you?" Helen and I say goodbye, and I promise her I will call the hospital at noon and see how Mother is doing.

Noon: I call the nurse's desk and am told Mother is now unresponsive. The doctor has been in and said she is in the final stages of death. I tell the nurse I probably can't be there before five and ask if I should try to get there sooner. "No," she says, "don't hurry."

And now this time seems final. After three months of good-bye and hello, I think this must be it. I call Don's office and ask them to locate him and tell him to come home immediately when his training session is over. Then I call John in Hope and ask him to go over so someone will be with her. Don cuts his training short and comes home and we leave.

3 P.M.: I am aware that this is the last time I will ever go back home to Mother. In the distance, through these hills of flint with their wind-bent grass, I see the road ending in the sky.

The hospital waits for us with its myriad healing colors. Bags of red and yellow, gleaming trays, and tubes with air lined up in impotent array beside my Mother.

I sit silently. Donavon is driving. It is a lonely prairie way, today. Nothing can make it bright. I see a solitary grain elevator far away, a hawk hangs just over the tall grass, there is a sign calling attention to the road construction on Highway 4 toward Hope. But Highway 4 is not my way anymore. I meet my past and see my future on the road going home to Mother this one last time.

5 P.M.: Don and I walk into the hospital room. I bend over to kiss Mother and she tries to say "I love you." The words are garbled, but I know them so well. I tell her John and I are there and Helen is on the way. I tell her I will be with her all the time now. She seems to understand and is not upset. A little later John decides to return to Hope because they are expecting guests for dinner and he has no way of contacting them. He looks at me and I can tell he is thinking there is still no telling how long this will take. We've been through this for three months. He leans over, kisses Mother, and tells her he will be back. Then, going out the door, he says, very loudly, "Goodbye Mother, Goodbye."

That final goodbye from John seems to be a signal to her. I think it is perhaps the last thing she understood other than feeling our love around her.

5:30 P.M.: Mother and I are alone. She stops breathing. I hold her hand and wait; I don't want anyone to intrude. Then I am overwhelmed with what is happening and I go out in the hall. One of the nurses, my cousin Jean, is there and I ask, "Will you please go get my husband?" Seeing my face, she comes in and checks on Mother. "Oh," she says, "she's gone." Then she notifies the nursing staff and goes to the waiting room to get Don. By the time Jean and Don return, Mother is breathing again.

Jean calls John at Hope just as he arrives in the door and tells him to come back. I know this is hard on Jean. All this summer, as we left at night, we were comforted when she was with Mother. Now she is comforting us again. She calls Reverend Okla to tell him what is happening.

In the meantime, Helen is on her way from Salina after getting her continuing education hours in a course on "Death and Dying." As she comes down the road from Hope to Herington she senses Mother is gone, but she sees John's car heading away from the hospital and it doesn't fit, so she assumes Mother is okay. When she gets to the hospital and sees my car, she expects the worst.

Helen comes in at 5:50 and sees me. She doesn't need an explanation. She begins to talk to Mother in that loving way only Helen has. She says, "It's all done now, Mama." She is telling her that it is okay. She is giving her permission to die.

Helen, who has been steady and caring for her these three rough months. Helen, who did not ask the "whys" like I did but just remained strong and able for her. I will never forget.

8 P.M.: Once again we children and our spouses are all gathered around Mother. The minister has been with us several hours. He has not intruded. He seems to be sorrowing also. Don and I go out and get something to eat. When we get back the others leave for the restaurant.

9:15 P.M.: Mother stops breathing again. Jean calls the restaurant, but by the time they get back, Mother is breathing. We stand and look at each other in amazement and the night wears on.

September 21

"Life is so short and love is so long."
Kasia Eryn Rutledge, age 11

Midnight: We decide that Helen and I will stay. John and
Maggie will go to Hope to rest, Tom to Durham, and Don
will rest in the waiting room. We will call them if there is
any change.

Helen has been up since 5 A.M., and she is sleepy but she
will not get in the other bed. I had promised Mother I would
watch with her. I tell Helen what I want to do, so she lies
down on the floor behind a chair and is soon fast asleep.

1 A.M.: A nurse comes in and tells Helen to get into the other
bed. I think Helen is too sleepy to protest and she does what
she is told. I have been sitting beside Mother all this time and
I now move to a more comfortable chair where I can watch
her. I see the rise and fall of her chest as she breathes, and I do
not believe she needs me beside her any longer. I do not think
she has been aware of anything since the first episode of
apnea.

2:30 A.M.: A nurse comes in to check on Mother. When she
leaves, she turns out the light. I intend to stay awake until
Helen has had some sleep and can relieve me, but I am so

very tired. Now in that darkened room, I listen to Mother's hoarse but even breathing, and I fall asleep.

3:00 A.M.: "Hey!" A loud, sharp voice calls out to me seemingly from high up in the room by the window. I sense something wrong. I struggle for wakefulness. I cannot hear Mother breathing! But I had promised her! I force my eyes to focus, remorse burning through my brain. I missed her passing. Finally I struggle from the chair and turn on the light.

I gently shake Helen, "It's over." She wakes instantly and we stand on either side of Mother. Helen removes the oxygen mask and closes the valve. I see beads of water on Mother's forehead and I reach down and touch the top of her head. It is very warm, almost hot, and the warmth is escaping. I look and look at her, expecting her to take a breath and she doesn't ever again. It is finally over. The dying is done.

Helen puts on the call light and the nurse comes in and does all those things nurses do when a person dies. She looks at her watch and says, "We'll set the death at 3:07." But I know better. At first I thought the voice that woke me was Mother's. Maybe I just wanted to think that. Perhaps it was my own. Some part of me was there in the room watching with her as I had said I would. And when the breathing stopped, I woke myself. Now I deeply regret my failure to sit with her through her last moments. Is this how the Disciples felt in Gethsemane when Jesus asked his sleeping followers why they could not have stayed awake that one last time? Almost instantly comes the thought that Mother would have understood my exhaustion.

John and Maggie have come back. I think Helen must have called them. Don is here, silent in the background. We children are waiting again in this room with our Mother. Only now it is oh so different. The feelings are flat. John says, "Today is Daddy's birthday." Maggie says, "Maybe that's the way she wanted it, so we could remember." No one cries. The sorrowing is very private right now. I look at Mother and see a mask and nothing else. I think to myself, death is really very ugly.

The funeral home has been called, and John tells us to go on, he will wait. We are all now suddenly aware of our tiredness, our own humanness. Still, I am torn about leaving this body that raged so against dying. Even though I know it cannot happen, I keep expecting her to start breathing again. But Helen has started outside to get into her car and it is a thirty-minute drive. I do not want her to go alone, so Don and I take our car and follow her. We leave Maggie Margaret and John to keep the last vigil.

In the car, I reach for my diary, and in the predawn darkness on the Lincolnville road, I write: September 21. Our Mother died today.

EPILOGUE

THE DIARY AFTER DEATH

Day 1

Morning comes early in the country. I woke to the smell of
coffee and the sounds of breakfast being made by Helen's
husband, Tom. We started making calls around 7 A.M. to tell
everyone that Mother had died four hours earlier and then
we went to Hope to make arrangements. The funeral home
attendants were genuinely supportive of us and respectful of
our privacy. But as they worked on Mother's obituary, it was
evident how little we remembered about her life. In the afternoon, Helen and I selected the family spray, a profusion of
baby's breath over fern, white carnations, and just a hint of
mauve daisies throughout. In the evening Donavon started
having chest pains, so we went back to the hospital. They ran
some tests and sent us back to Topeka to get some rest. By
then we were very tired. I remember stopping at a filling station in Junction City and telling the attendant that Mother
died today. I wanted to tell it to everyone I met. It was not
for sympathy. It was more like trying it on to see if it fit. If
I could say it, maybe it would feel real.

Day 2

We spent the day preparing clothes and making more phone
calls. Kirk met Aunt Helen at the airport in Kansas City and

brought her to Topeka for us. That evening we went to the Hunam Restaurant and celebrated Kirk's belated birthday dinner. It was a strange day. I felt as if I should be at Hope, yet there was no reason to be. There always was a Mother at Hope and now there is just Hope and a little cottage and a very strange feeling like something isn't quite right in Hope.

Day 3

In the morning, Donavon, Aunt Helen, and I drove to Hope to the funeral home. I had told the funeral director that Mother never wore makeup and not to put color on her face. Isabell, the hairdresser who had set her 1920-style fingertip wave for over fifteen years, had fixed her hair in those pretty waves that were so uniquely hers. But as I looked at her, I realized that I had never paid close attention to her physical features. All I ever looked for on her face was love and caring. That was gone and that was what I wanted to see. This person looked like a stranger, like a prim and proper schoolteacher. Helen had selected a blue skirt and ruffled white long-sleeved blouse for her. She would have been glad that Helen told her what to wear on her last time to get "dressed up." She had never liked worrying about what to wear.

We then went to John's. The neighbors had brought in food, so there was plenty to eat. In the evening we went to the family service at the funeral home. There was a pleasing array of flowers. Our spray looked nice with the bronze casket and its natural-color drapes. There were about twenty-five people there from Helen's little country church. It was obvious they loved Helen. Mother's whole life was built around her devotion to her religion, and her beliefs never wavered. That was often hard to deal with, but after she died, Donavon told me something that helped comfort me. He said, "In spite of her rigid adherence to her beliefs, when it came down to dealing with others, in every instance, Mom was a humane and loving person and made the right decisions." Her humanity was evident that night. Over forty years ago one of my cousins fell in love with a young woman of another faith. Neither family approved of the other. They went to Mother for support, and even though she shared some of the same religious prejudices, she was able to give them comfort and advice. They married, raised a lovely family, did well financially, and are still married. On this evening, they came a long distance to say their good-byes to Mother.

Mother's old neighbor from across the street was there. He came in out of breath and hardly able to walk, and I wonder if he is surprised that she went first. He said, "We thought a lot of your Mother." Then I heard him murmur under his breath, ". . . every day she went to the post office, every Sunday she went to church . . . every day to the post office . . . every Sunday to church . . ." Berniece, Mother's friend who had worked with her for many years, was there. She said, "I learned so much from your Mother. One day I had forgotten to get something important done. Alice didn't say anything, just went ahead and did it, but I know she was irritated. Finally I said to her, 'Alice, I intended to do it.' Your Mother turned to me and said, 'The road to hell is paved with good intentions.'" When I told Helen about it, later that evening, Helen marveled, "Mama must have really been mad."

Reverend Okla presided over a brief service. He said that Mother had never lost her faith or her sense of humor. He said that when he first went to the hospital and was introduced as the new minister, her eyes just lit up because the church at Hope was her main concern. He closed with scripture and prayer. We had a late supper at John's and went to Helen's to sleep for a few hours.

Day 4

Leaving Helen's home 3 miles west of Durham in Marion County, take Highway 15 north for 13 miles. At Elmo, in Dickinson County, turn east and follow Highway 4 around the curves and over the hills toward Hope. Relatives and friends live along this road. Pass the graveyard and the Anderson farm. Now the land evens out and you will see the water tower in the distance. HOPE.

It is a bright prairie day. The dying grasses wave gently, the soft white clouds are back. Our new car, with thousands of miles of prairie driving on the odometer, smoothly sets the pace for the others behind us. Time is standing still. This is Tuesday and people should be at work. There are cousins and aunts and uncles here who should be somewhere else. We are all suspended in this place. The earth is motionless. Perhaps tomorrow, time will return.

The Funeral

In the church basement, women of the church have prepared lunch for the seventy-five relatives here. While we are eating, Mother's casket and flowers are brought into the sanctuary above us. We go up one last time before everyone arrives. Kasia cried and then described her feelings: "As I stood there looking down at Greatgrandmother laying there, I found myself hoping that I would see her chest heave and see her speak. But she just lay there leaving me with nothing but a puddle of memories . . ." Eight-year-old Jennifer Dru was her same Dru self. When she heard that Greatgrandmother's body was upstairs, she asked, "How did they get her here?" Donavon said, "She came in the hearse." Dru began to sing, "Whenever you see a hearse go by . . ." Donavon stopped her, saying that the song wasn't appropriate. "Why?" she asked. Later during the service she drew a picture of a heart torn in two. The verse underneath it read, "In sorrow we will weep, but our love we'll always keep."

I think of the first Memorial Day after my Father died. There was a little boy in Hope who loved Mother and often showed up for a chat and a cookie. One day he asked her, "Where is your Daddy [husband]?" Mother explained that he had died and was buried in the cemetery two blocks away. The little boy went and found Daddy's grave. It was two days before Memorial Day and there were flowers on all the graves but none yet on Dan Brunner's. The peonies Mother had cut before they bloomed were sitting in a jar in the refrigerator. He did not know this. He simply saw an undecorated grave.

The next day, Mother took her peonies to decorate Daddy's grave. As she walked across the grass, she was horrified. There was not a single flower on any grave except Daddy's, and it was completely covered with flowers! In the morning there would be veterans and flags, and the townsfolk who had already decorated would turn out. Mother, not knowing where the wreaths belonged, took them off Daddy's grave and placed them alongside the lane. The next day at dinner, she told us. We laughed and reminded her that nobody would enjoy that story more than Daddy. But Mother never did laugh about it.

Before the service, Mother's casket was open at the back of the church. People had the option of going by or not while our cousin, the Reverend Eugene Hicks, played a selection of classical music on the organ. When it was time for the service, the casket was closed and sealed and the family followed it to the front.

Sunlight filtered through the windows into the old church with its polished wooden pews and yellow wood floor, as we followed Mother on her last trip into this place that had been so large a part of her life. Most of her significant life passages were marked here and now we were at her single most important event.

The Riffels sang "Morning Has Broken" by Eleanor Farjeon and I thought about the people who had come. I resisted my impulse to turn and look at their faces, to see how they had loved our Mother. During the singing of Mother's favorite hymn, "Precious Lord," I thought of the many times she had sung it, and it was never so appropriate as now. "I am tired, I am weak, I am worn . . . take my hand . . . lead me home."

Rev. Okla Gawith conducted the service, and Mother's nephew Ray Stites, president of Nebraska Christian College, gave a brief message. In it, he explained how we cousins were raised and what our heritage meant to him. He said that as a child, he didn't know there were people who never went to church. He recalled a Sunday morning when the cattle got out, he and his dad got them back in, and then showed up in church as they were singing the last hymn.

Ray reminded us that Mother's people had been a part of this church and community for over a century, and at least three family members entered the ministry. I can remember hearing my uncles tell how the first generation of Anderson men would sit in the back row at church, and if the preacher talked too long, they would pull out their big pocket watches and wind them!

When Ray referred to Mother as "Aunt Al," we all laughed because that was John's favorite way to tease Mother. Helen and I never dared to use it, but John was incorrigible. When she was in her late sixties, working at a care-home for the aged, John would ask, "Well Al, how were the inmates today?" And she would just shake her head. Ray, describing our family's penchant for laughing through misfortune, said, "There are a lot of humorists in this family, many humorists in fact. They're not always funny, but they're humorists."

The scripture Ray used was one Mother had underscored again and again in her Bible. From Corinthians, it was an explanation of having sorrow and yet joy, turmoil and yet peace, ending with, "having nothing and yet possessing everything."

Reverend Okla sang "The Lord's Prayer," and several of the grandchildren participated in the service. Debbie said, "I first met Grandma when I was four . . ." and told of how she had been accepted. Joel, in an emotion-laden voice, explained how Grandma always talked about Jesus as though she had just come in from a walk in the garden with Him. Kasia read a poem, ". . . Slowly His soft kind voice whispered in your ear (and) you entered the land of rest . . . I will always remember you . . ." The youngest child from each family, Christina, Joel, and Joy, read "I'll Love You Forever" by Robert Munsch. This simple story of a love that spanned generations had comforted Mother and all of us this past year.

The last song was one I had often sung for Mother, "Many things about tomorrow I don't seem to understand. But I know who holds tomorrow and I know who holds my hand." After the closing prayer, and while Gene played "Come, Ye Disconsolate," we followed the casket outside. It was carried by her youngest cousin, Jim Anderson, and five of her nephews, Jack, Ashley, and Tom Anderson, Lauren Brunner, and Lee Kaiser. We passed through an honor guard of elderly churchmen.

199

The Burial

Turn north at the first corner east of the church. Go 1 block, turn right. The second house on the left side of the street is Mother's cottage. Continue 3 more blocks past the school's baseball field, John's house, and beyond the edge of town. You can't miss it. This road ends in the cemetery.

Just a short drive now and it's almost over. We follow the streets through this dusty little Kansas town, past the cottage we know so well, kicking up road dust until we turn onto the grassy drive of the cemetery. I wonder how many times had Mother come to this place since Daddy died? I remember Mother's and Grandmother's time-honored tradition of decorating all the graves in May. Who is there now to tend the graves of those whose names we no longer speak? Who is there to know that the Andersons are buried west of town, the Robinsons north, the Brunners and Grandpa Beisel south?

Time, which stood still less than four hours ago, is now flying. I strain to hold these final moments with me a little longer. I hesitate, get slowly out of the car. And then, there we are, sitting on velvet-covered chairs with wind whipping the metal on the ends of the cords against the metal legs of the canopy, creating a soft tinkle and an occasional crash against the background of the very brief ashes to ashes, dust to dust service. We huddle closely against the wind in order to hear.

The wind has come to say goodbye. It touches my face, pushes against my back, lifts my hair, then dances over to ruffle the flowers on Mother's casket. She knew this wind. For seventy-nine years it accompanied her to the clothesline. Tossed dust at her in the garden. Picked up strands of her hair and flung them around. Blew her Sunday hat into the mud and her gardening hat into the water tank. And it had sent fresh air and foul into her kitchen whenever it pleased. The wind will be back tomorrow and the tomorrow after that. It will blow leaves and dust as it has every fall, and soon, in the coming winter, it will blow snow across . . . her.

I turn to the people around us. And then I realize that the voices are all saying the same thing. Mother had meant much to them and they would miss her. They did not just shake our hands and tell us they were sorry for us. It was themselves they were sorry for.

We drive the short distance to John's house and talk about getting together next week to write thank-you notes. I know there are going to be some painful days ahead. I will wish I could talk to her, but we had a whole life of quality time. Aunt Helen reminds me that if something goes on forever, do we really know its value?

Day 5

"Life . . . a shadow which runs across the grass . . ."
Crowfoot, 1890

All the relatives have gone back to what they were doing before the intrusion of Mother's death into their lives. I am filled with chaotic feelings. They do not surprise me, and all day I try to be aware, for I know change comes out of chaos and healing will come from accepting change.

But the balance has shifted. I felt it go in her room the night she died. I am walking carefully, not getting too close to the edge. Mother's death seems to float along the edges of this time I have put boundaries on. There is movement, but where will the movement end?

I spend most of the day wondering how to feel. In late afternoon, panic builds in me. Around five o'clock I begin to cry. This is the time of day when the school bus got home from school. This is the dinner hour when we gathered around the table. This is the time for worrying about family members who do not make it home.

And the one person on this earth who would love me no matter how bad I was, no matter how I disappointed her, no *matter what,* will never again wait to welcome us all home, to nurture us, to make it well. Never again. No matter I had not needed her strength for thirty years. No matter it was I who gave her support in recent years. What mattered was it would never be again.

In the midst of my loneliness, I remember the comforting words of Crowfoot, an orator from the Blackfoot Tribe, which

Daniel whispered to me at the graveside. As Crowfoot lay dying in 1890, his last words were of life.

> What is life? It is the flash of a firefly in the night. It is the breath of a buffalo in the wintertime. It is the little shadow which runs across the grass and loses itself in the sunset.

And that is how it was for Alice Anderson Brunner. Mother's life was filled with friends and relatives and love and caring events. But in the wholeness of time, she was a little shadow that ran across the tall-grass hills and disappeared into the sunset that had given her so much comfort. I turn my mind to the hills and the sky and I am again comforted.

Day 14

> A day in which I push out the boundaries of my life.

Fall is the time of year Mother loved the best. It is a time of sadness, of introspection. So I marvel at how I accepted Mother's death. The things I had been worried about simply did not happen. Instead, it was a time to find out just how strong I was. And there is no doubt in my mind from whom I got strength.

I have tried to be faithful to Mother's beliefs in this diary. I no longer question or care to question my Mother's faith. That was part of my youth, and I am comfortable with where I am and with where she was. So, on the morning she died, as Donavon and I drove into the rising sun, I could truthfully say, "I trust Mother finds exactly what she intended to find today."

I am holding an empty envelope addressed to Mother. It is from our Park Place address in Wichita, so it is at least three years old. I look at it and I wonder what it was I did not send? What it was I intended to say? It is so unfinished. Something forever unsaid.

At my desk now, watching the trees outside lose their leaves, feeling rays from the morning sun on my back, I feel Mother's presence beside me. It has come quietly and spread over me and I am immersed in warmth. There is no touch, only a presence of energy centered in this room. It is a concentration of love so pure nothing can obscure it. No maybes. No hidden agendas. None of the old strife. Just love. If I look around, she will be there. But there is no need to look. The presence is Mother. I am calm and I am oh so warm and whole and comforted.

I do not know how long I sit with her presence near me. But now, the thinking part of me intrudes, shouting to me a realization of what has just happened and from whom it came. Here I am with the knowledge that love transcends death!

Her body is gone, but her love remains. I have just discovered enormous power. Nothing I know is more powerful than this love. I feel a sense of triumph at the discovery. Mother had the power of love. Do I have it, too?

It is over. I have focused on myself and missed the movement outside of me. Still, a memory of warmth remains while I begin to call my children. Both Lance and Daniel are out of their offices, but I reach Joel and Doni Marie. "Do you know what I just discovered?" I try to explain it, but it is unexplainable. "I felt her presence . . . I felt her love . . . I just discovered love does not die and you can feel love when the person who loved you is dead!" Like me, Joel tries to intellectualize it. Doni gently asks, "Did you call me to tell me this?" And then I realize they can't possibly understand. It is outside of their experience, and mine, too, until an hour ago.

On this day, I let go of the old paradigms and pushed the center out of the boundaries of my life. In doing so, I found death cannot remove, destroy, or otherwise change love. Death has no final effect on love. I have been face to face with the power of love.

Day 30

It has been a month since Mother's death. John, Helen, and I are preparing for the holiday season in our own ways with our own families. There is now no generation between us and death, and so we stand face to face with our own mortality. And Mother? Mother has changed. The energy that was her body has been used up and her spirit remains.

Most of us fear dying. But I took the gift Mother gave me, of opening my eyes and looking at nothing until I saw everything. By dealing with her death in that manner, I was no longer at the mercy of my emotions.

But for some of the people who loved our Mother, the fear of death became larger than their passion for living. So they came to her death not realizing she was going on in a different form, just seeing the end of the old. Hospital personnel, friends, ministers, and doctors quaked at the prospect of death. It was something they did not understand, so life was to be prolonged as long as possible—at all costs. Throughout time, people have attempted to explain death by placing limits upon it, but they have succeeded only in creating mass confusion and collective fear.

Author Merle Bird once told me that death is a mystery and that you don't explain mysteries, you just accept them. With Mother, I walked into and through my fear of death. It was a privileged gift. And now, because I have been on a journey that few choose, the world looks different. I see some things clearly for the first time. I know everything I've done or will do is shared; everyone I've touched or will touch is remembered; my being here will be carried on through time by love.

During her final years on the prairie, when suffering and loneliness had become a large part of her life, Mother shared with us how she struggled to overcome feelings of uselessness. She would wake in the morning thinking, "If I can just be of some use to someone," and go to sleep in the evening feeling she had failed. This past winter, on a cheerful, happy day, she said to me, "Now I know there is some reason why I am here. I have yet to be of some help to someone!"

Today I know she found that "way to be of use to someone." And I know for whom she did it. It was for me. She showed me how to die. See you in the morning, Mother.

THE BEGINNING

FINAL ENTRY
FROM THE DIARY

June 6, 1992

In the summer after Mother died, I asked Joel to read my
diary. I wanted him to tell me whether or not I had captured
the essence of Mother and been true to her faith. When Joel
was finished with the manuscript, he tacked a note onto it.
This affirmation of love is my final entry in this Diary of
Dying and Living on the Kansas Prairie.

> Mom,
>
> I loved my Grandma very much.
> I know too, that Grandma loved me.
> She loved so many people
> and was loved in return.
> My images of Grandma are beautifully kept
> in the pages of this diary
> and I pray as she would have wanted me to,
> for these words to be a comfort to others.
> I know they will.
> Grandma loves you, too!
>
> Joel

Why would anyone keep a diary of the death of a woman
who never made the front page of a newspaper, who had no

money, who did not climb a social ladder, who never wrote any books, sang any songs, painted any pictures, and who is buried in a small, out-of-the-way prairie town where she was born and lived out her life?

The answer is in this final entry. Even as her grandson recognized and affirmed the power of her love, so do I. Love is all that matters.

ALICE OF HOPE

Alice was born March 11, 1912, to John Anderson and Clara Robinson. She had two sisters and two brothers, Edna, Helen, Orville, and Howard.

John's father, Charles, had come to America from Sweden just two generations before, while Clara's ancestors came as Pilgrims to a new and unexplored world in the 1600s. By the late 1800s, both families had homesteaded near Hope, Kansas, the Robinsons to the east of town and the Andersons to the west. They were about equal distances from the heart of town.

At the time of Alice's birth, her grandfather Robinson was a justice of the peace who performed marriages and settled disputes among community folks. He had a large library that Alice used from the time she could read. Alice, when a youth, was baptized in the Hope Christian church. She went by horse and buggy to school in Hope and graduated from high school in 1930. At age eighteen, she passed the teacher's examination and began to teach in a one-room school near Council Grove in the heart of the Flint Hills. She then taught at two other rural schools, but her career as a teacher was short-lived. At Rosebank, some pupils brought their uncle, Daniel Brunner, to meet this pretty, dark-eyed teacher.

Daniel Brunner and Alice Anderson were married on the Anderson farm near Hope. After a brief honeymoon in Colorado, they settled south of Hope on the old Eisenhower place where their children were born, John Daniel in 1936, Carol Marie in 1938, and Helen Rose in 1939. In 1940 the family moved to Illinois, returning in five years to a farm near the Marion/Dickinson county line. Those brief years near Sugar Grove, Illinois, marked the only time Dan and Alice lived outside the Hope community.

When their children were raised and gone from home, and when Dan's eyesight failed, they moved from the farm to a little cottage in Hope. There Alice worked as a cook for fifteen years in the Hope schools, enjoying all the children with whom she came in touch. She later became a clerk in Lloyd's Grocery.

During this time, John and his wife, Margaret Fowler, were raising Debra, Richard, Russell, Roger, Robert, and Christina in the Abilene community. Richard died when he was nineteen years old. Carol and her husband, Donavon Rutledge, were raising Lance, Daniel, Doni Marie, and Joel in the Wichita community. Helen and her husband, Tom Bishop, were raising Robin, Alyce, and Joy in West Virginia, eventually returning to Marion County, Kansas.

When Dan died in 1980, Alice went to work as an aide at the Lutheran Home in Herington until a heart condition kept her from working.

The family was growing. Greatgrandchildren now included
Jeremy, Josh, Kasia, Jennifer Dru, Lacey, Tahnoqua, Travis, Nichole, Cody, Taiomah, and Tyler.

Alice died September 21, 1991. She and Dan were born, reared, married, bore their children, raised their family, grew to old age, and died in the little community around Hope in Dickinson County, Kansas. Simple stones mark their graves in the Hope cemetery.

FOR THE READER

Take Kansas Highway 4 out to the rim of the prairie or travel the high road along Skyline Drive to where the hills flow into each other and the wind constantly moves.

If the space feels different than it ever has before. If you see a hawk balanced on top of a high place. If you notice the grasses bending a certain direction. If you see a tree and wonder why it is there. If you stand alone in the prairie sea and hear the whisperings of tall grass. If you have a sense that none of it and all of it is yours. And if, in the early morning or late evening light, you are privileged to see purple in the hills—then you will have seen my prairie.